Body Rx

Body

A. Scott Connelly, M.D.,
and Carol Colman

G. P. Putnam's Sons   *New York*

Dr. Scott Connelly's 6-Pack Prescription

R_x

6 Meals a Day

6 Weeks to Strength

6 Weeks to Sculpt

6 Weeks to Burn Fat

6 Weeks to Maintain

———————————————

= **6** Months to a Great Body

G. P. Putnam's Sons
Publishers Since 1838
a member of
Penguin Putnam Inc.
375 Hudson Street
New York, NY 10014

Library of Congress Cataloging-in-Publication Data

Connelly, A. Scott.
    Body Rx : Dr. Scott Connelly's 6-pack prescription /
A. Scott Connelly and Carol Colman.
        p.   cm.
    Includes bibliographical references.
    ISBN 0-399-14782-9
    1. Health.   2. Physical fitness.   3. Nutrition.
    4. Exercise.   I. Colman, Carol.   II. Title.
RA776 C758   2001   2001019729
613—dc21

Printed in the United States of America

10   9   8   7   6   5   4   3   2   1

This book is printed on acid-free paper. ∞

Book design by Lee Fukui
Exercise photographs by Nick Vaccaro
Photographs of Jason Sehorn before: Gary Hillstead; Dottie
Lessard-O'Connor before: Beverly Lessard; after: Karen
Couture; Deb Klipper before: David Klipper; after:
Billy Carpenter

Acknowledgments

First and foremost, we'd like to thank everyone at Penguin Putnam, from the publisher to the publicity department to the sales force, who has shaped this project, nurtured it, and brought it into the world. In particular, we'd like to thank our amazing editor, Jeremy Katz, who transformed the book, and himself in the process. It was a pleasure working with him. A big thank you to Sharon Lindsey, a brilliant publicist, and Mike Danielson of Media Relations, who helped launch the project by putting Scott in touch with Carol. It has been a wonderful collaboration. Many thanks to Linda York, who put Scott in touch with his agent, Ellen Geiger, her assistant, Anna Abreu, and the wonderful team at Curtis Brown. A warm thank you to Carol's agent, Richard Curtis, for his enthusiasm and support. We would also like to express a debt of gratitude to Billy Carpenter for his hard work, and Deb Klipper for serving as an exercise model. Many thanks to Jason Sehorn and Dottie Lessard-O'Connor for sharing their stories.

PRINTING HOUSE
FITNESS AND RACQUET CLUB

A special thank you to New York City's Printing House gym for the use of its facilities for the exercise photographs in this book.

To my father, Clinton A. Connelly,
who always encouraged me to embrace opportunities
and seek my true potential regardless of the obstacles in my path

Contents

Body Rx

How would you like to have a great body—the kind of body you never dreamed you could have?

If that sounds inviting, then this book is required reading. The fitness and fat-loss program outlined here will show you how to change your body composition, radically. What is body composition? It's the ratio of lean body mass to fat mass, and as you can well imagine, it's lean body mass you want. Moreover, *Body Rx* can teach you how to burn off fat without depleting lean body tissue. Other diets chew up the beneficial parts of the body in order to bring about weight loss.

I've devoted the past three decades of my life to the science of metabolism. From my earliest days studying and researching at Harvard and Stanford, I've been investigating how the human body uses nutrients. I've studied how we make fat, how we burn fat, how we make muscle, and how we stay in shape. I've put my research to work in the intensive care unit, helping dreadfully ill patients return to health. And I've put my research to work also helping elite athletes, bodybuilders, and the fitness-conscious achieve peak performance. And now you can put it to work for yourself.

Before you dive into this program, here are some tips to make the Body Rx 6-Pack Prescription work for you:

- *Don't count calories.* I know you've heard that before, but this program is not about calorie deprivation. On my program you'll probably be eating more calories than you ever have eaten before. And you'll be eating satisfying foods like dairy, meats, fruits, and vegetables.

- *Get off the treadmill.* My exercise philosophy revolves around strength training. You get all the benefits—even the healthy-heart benefits—of aerobics from strength training, in addition to a lean, sculpted body that is impossible to achieve on aerobics alone.

- *Tailor this program to fit your needs.* I've set up my program to work for you even if you follow only part of it. While I love exercise (I am as comfortable in the weight room as I am in the operating room), I have to level with you: You can get seventy percent of the benefit of the Body Rx 6-Pack Prescription from the nutrition program alone. If you know right now that there is no way you will ever step into a gym, don't even bother to read the chapters on exercise. Instead, read the chapters on nutrition two or three times.

- *A note to women:* Our culture bombards you with destructive messages. Obsessive calorie counting, endless aerobics, and insane dieting advice have contributed to an epidemic of obesity.

Women must pay attention to muscle and metabolism and start thinking differently about their bodies.

- *Even if you listen to nothing else, listen to me on fructose.* Over the past twenty years, the degeneration of our food supply brought on by industrialization has dramatically accelerated. As the obesity epidemic grows, the changes that have been made in our food supply have outpaced our ability to adapt metabolically. While it is tempting to blame a sedentary life or out-of-control eating habits, the truth is simpler. Our eating behavior has remained basically the same. So what's the problem? The food supply is no longer appropriate for our bodies. I believe the key problem is a ubiquitous additive that has invaded our food supply over the past two decades: fructose. Even if you listen to nothing else I say, read and reread the fructose chapter. The tiny changes it recommends will make a huge difference to your body composition.

As a physician, I had the responsibility to save the lives of patients in my care. As I expanded my work out of the hospital and into the world at large, my mission grew. I discovered that the lives I can save in the operating room are just a fraction of those I can save in the world at large. I'm a metabolism scientist with one foot in the medical world and one in the weight room. I want to teach you what I've learned from both arenas. As a physician, I'm going to offer you a prescription for optimum nutrition. As your trainer, I'm going to whip you into shape. As a result, you're going to have the body you never dreamed you could have.

My goal is to transform *Body Rx* into a book with no ending, and to provide each and every reader with direct access to me and other experts and teachers. To find out more about this wealth of additional information, log on to www.bodyrxinfo.com or call 1-877-226-3979 (1-877-2BODYRX).

Part I

Throw Out Your Scale

1

If you shudder at just the *thought* of being seen in public in a bathing suit—if you can't stand looking at yourself naked in the mirror—you're in good company. Recently, I received a frantic call from a well-known actress, who, for reasons that will soon be apparent, I am not going to name.

She was desperate to book as many training sessions as she could as soon as possible. While I scrolled through my calendar, trying to find dates when I could squeeze her in, I asked her my standard question:

"What are your goals?"

She explained that in a few weeks she had to film a brief nude scene.

The thought of taking her clothes off for the camera was more than she could bear.

"I don't even like to undress in front of a mirror," she confessed. "I want to look better naked."

Her answer resonated with me, as it probably does with you. Think about it. When was the last time you stood in front of the mirror—stark naked—and thought, *Hey, I look great*?

When was the last time you actually looked forward to putting on a bathing suit or trying on clothes?

When was the last time you felt really good about your body?

And, more important, when was the last time you felt really good *in* your body?

Perhaps you're thinking, *Never!* Perhaps you're thinking, *Not since I was 19*. It doesn't matter. All of that is about to change. In *Body Rx*, I will show you how to make your body strong, sculpted, and lean. For the first time in years—maybe for the first time in your life—you will like what you see in the mirror. You can have the body you want.

Body Rx teaches you a dramatically new way of thinking about how and what to eat. It introduces you to my 6-Pack Prescription, an innovative approach to nutrition and fitness that has given thousands of people the bodies they've always wanted. I'm not just talking to those of you who want to lose a few pounds or want to do a little bodily tuning up. *Body Rx* will bring about dramatic transformations for men and women who have been fighting a lifelong losing battle with obesity, discouraged dieters who have spent years counting calories and growing fat, baby boomers seeking to stave off middle-age spread, and even superstar athletes, such as New York Giants cornerback Jason Sehorn and future Hall of Fame pitcher Roger Clemens (both of whom have trained with me) . . . and yes, even actresses (and actors) shaping up for the occasional nude scene.

Body Rx is cutting-edge science based on my work as a physician and researcher. It introduces you to the recent breakthroughs in the study of metabolism that have finally revealed the secret to having a slim, attractive, healthy body without starving yourself, cutting calories, or using dangerous drugs. The same research has answered questions that perplexed scientists (and dieters!) have had for decades: why those who eat the least often weigh the most; why diets fail 90 percent of the time; why Americans are growing fatter every year; and why maintaining a trim, attractive body has become a major life struggle for most Americans, even our children.

I am a doctor, but not a diet doctor. My areas of speciality are critical care, metabolism, and cardiovascular anesthesiology. Mostly, I think of myself as an inventor. Some years ago I developed a special protein formula that is used in critical-care units of hospitals all over the world to keep severely ill patients from wasting to death. I'm proud of how many lives it has saved. The protein formula I developed to treat patients is also the main ingredient in a sports nutrition product called Met-Rx that I later developed for bodybuilders and other athletes. In the course of creating that formula and in the ten years since then, I researched the principles of metabolism and protein that are the foundation of *Body Rx*'s 6-Pack Prescription.

6-pack is the term that athletes and weight lifters have long used to describe well-defined abdominal muscles. Today men and women of all ages know and use the term to describe one of their primary fitness goals. In fact, in Hollywood a 6-pack is the newest status symbol. But the significance of the 6-pack extends far beyond the cosmetic. A 6-pack is a sign of a strong, healthy body with good muscle tone. It is a sign of a body that is less likely to succumb to obesity, heart disease, diabetes, and the many other diseases that run rampant through our aging, overweight population. Believe it or not, a 6-pack is a goal everyone can achieve.

My 6-Pack Prescription is composed of four six-week cycles, each of which has a different eating plan, weight-training program, and optional supplement regimen that work synergistically to produce maximum results. This is not a meal plan or exercise program that you have heard before. On the meal plan, you will be full and satisfied, eating more than you dreamed possible. On the weight-training regimen, your body will be transformed weekly without hours of endless aerobics. As you follow the meal plan, you will see palpable change in your body composition. You will build muscle at the expense of your fat, adding shape and tone to your body. As you follow the workout, even more extraordinary changes will occur. During Cycle 1, "6 Weeks to Strength," you will get stronger. During Cycle 2, "6 Weeks to Sculpt," you will use your improved strength to make more muscle, creating a more sculpted, defined appearance. During Cycle 3, "6 Weeks to Burn Fat," you will put this new muscle to work burning fat and getting leaner. During Cycle 4, "6 Weeks to Maintenance and Endurance," you will follow a maintenance program that will get you started on staying slim and lean for life. By the end of twenty-four weeks, your metabolism will be significantly transformed, and so will your body. You *will* look better naked! But you will also be stronger, healthier, and happier than you have been in years.

Unlike all the other programs out there, the goal of the 6-Pack Prescription is to transform your body into something you'll be proud of for the rest of your life. While nutrition can take you a long way toward that goal, my exercise prescription will help get you the rest of the way. The 6-Pack Prescription is scientifically designed to build high-quality muscle that burns fat better and faster than anything else. You don't have to work out for hours every day to get this great result. Give me four hours a week and I can transform your body.

Although I do recommend the use of a few nutrition supplements, I want to make it clear that supplements are optional. You can still achieve fantastic results without them. I recommend products only generically so that you can purchase any brands that are most convenient and economical.

I Walk the Walk

I practice what I preach, and it shows. I am in great shape. I am six foot five, weigh 230 pounds, and look great, because I have less than 5 percent body fat. I do have a 6-pack. Not bad for a guy of 50! I don't mean to boast: I'm telling you this for an important reason.

I don't think one should be in the business of giving people this kind of advice unless he not only "talks the talk" but "walks the walk." Have you noticed how many self-proclaimed diet doctors look unfit? Why anyone would or should take nutritional advice from people who look so bad eludes me. I recently challenged several of the top diet gurus to a televised debate. My only requirement was that everyone wear a bathing suit. Not one of these so-called diet experts was willing to show his or her body in public. What are they hiding? Not their 6-packs! When I tell you that my program works, you don't have to take my word for it: You can see it.

Through the years, I have worked with a number of celebrities and superstar athletes, but I've also helped train lots of regular folks whom I meet at the Met-Rx Gym. I've also consulted with fitness trainers throughout the country on their more difficult cases, but the most rewarding part of my work is seeing how my approach to fitness and nutrition has transformed both the bodies and the lives of thousands of men and women. Feeling in control of your body spills over into other aspects of your life. When you are proud of yourself, you exude the confidence of someone who is on the right track. You know that you can do more and achieve more in every area of your life. In other words, you project charisma—and I've seen it happen time and time again. So that's why I'm proud of my body: It is a constant reminder to me of the thousands of people who have joined me in becoming their best selves.

Despite the scores of popular diet books published in the last couple of decades—or perhaps because of them—Americans have grown fatter and fatter.

In 1980, 30 percent of all American adults were seriously overweight; *today, more than half are*. A shocking 13 percent of our children and teenagers are severely overweight, despite the natural tendency of children to be lean. And those same fat children are much more likely to grow into fat adults.

For the past twenty years, the universal prescription for obesity has been a weight-loss diet. Each diet has its own gimmick, but the bottom line is the same. When all is said and done, you are attempting to shed pounds by drastically cutting calories. Great. That must work, right?

Wrong. Take a look around you. Half the population is still fat.

Despite all this wonderful advice, half the population is overweight and getting fatter by the minute. Why? All of these diets are based on antiquated notions about food and weight loss! None addresses the underlying cause of obesity, and so the "fat epidemic" rages out of control.

Are You a Fat Storage Machine?

Before you can understand why everyone is getting fatter, you need to know about metabolism. Metabolism is the way your body breaks down and uses the nutrients it derives from food. At one time scientists and physicians generally believed that one metabolic rule applied to everyone: that regardless of who we are and what we eat, our bodies burn whatever calories they need for energy, and store the excess as fat. Thus, those of us who consume too many calories store too much fat, and get fat.

Not exactly.

Today a growing number of scientists and physicians—I am one of them—reject this one-size-fits-all approach to nutrition. We think it tells only half the story.

We have identified another force at work within the body—a critical phenomenon that we call nutrient partitioning—that affects how our bodies handle the food we consume. It's a phenomenon that can either work for us or against us. Let me explain.

There are two different ways that nutrients are handled in the body after they are broken down or metabolized. They can be burned for energy, or they can be stored. If they are stored, they are stored either as fat deposits or lean mass, which is mostly muscle. We humans are born with a metabolic tendency to be either *fat burners* or *fat storers*. Fat burners are fortunate. They have a natural tendency to burn body fat and store muscle. They can get away with eating almost anything without suffering the consequences. The rest of us—about two thirds of the population—have a natural tendency to burn muscle and store fat. We are fat storers. Now, this doesn't mean that we're born to be fat—not at all! All it means is that our bodies are predisposed to hoard fat and burn other nutrients for energy.

Why are so many of us fat storers? Because our ancestors were, and had to be. Long ago, when food was scarce and famine was a very real threat, the ability to store fat was an asset. It enabled our ancestors to survive. Indeed, had our ancestors not been fat storers, we might not be here today to complain about it! But of course, times have changed. Now that food is abundant, the tendency to store fat is no longer an evolutionary edge. On the contrary, it can be harmful. Our ancestors stored fat because they had to. We store fat whether we have to or not, and nutrient partitioning is to blame.

Think of nutrient partitioning as a metabolic traffic cop directing nutrient traffic into one of two parking lots. Nutrients that he directs to the lot on the right are parked as muscle or lean body mass. Nutrients that he directs to the lot on the left are parked as fat. (I will provide more information on nutrient partitioning in Chapter 2, "The Metabolic Meltdown.") While the natural fat burners get off easy, the rest of us must be careful to keep our metabolic traffic cop happy. Unfortunately, some of the foods we eat confuse our metabolic traffic cops, interfering with their ability to direct nutrient flow. As a result, too many nutrients are parked at fat. Some of the most common ingredients in the food supply are the worst offenders.

Our modern diet is filled with foods and additives that drive the metabolic traffic cop to shunt too many nutrients into the fat parking lot. Scientists call them *negative partitioning agents*. To compound the problem, we have reduced our consumption and in some cases eliminated many of the foods that keep the metabolic traffic cop running smoothly—the *positive partitioning agents*.

The focus of the 6-Pack Prescription Meal Plan is on nutrient partitioning, *not calorie counting*. I am more concerned about the *quality* of the food that you eat than the *quantity*. If your diet is filled with foods that are positive partitioning agents, you can eat to your heart's delight and not get fat. If your diet is filled with foods that are negative partitioning agents, you can starve yourself and still be fat.

As the Body Inflates, the Ego Deflates

When your fat-storage switch is turned on, it's difficult to feel good about your body. Excess body fat is what makes you look (and feel) fat, dumpy, and unattractive. Excess body fat is what makes your waist expand annually and what makes trying on a bathing suit so agonizing.

But diet, exercise, and drugs per se are not the answer. Unless you turn the fat-storage switch off and the fat burning switch on—unless you instruct your metabolic traffic cop to divert nutrients away from the fat parking lot and into the muscle and lean mass parking lot—you can count calories until the cows come home and you can run on the treadmill until you topple over, but you will not get the results you want.

To change how you look on the outside, you need to reverse what's happening on the inside. You need to reprogram your body to burn fat and manufacture muscle and lean mass. Muscle is what makes you look slim, sleek, and well proportioned. Muscle is what makes you feel good about your body. Muscle is what makes you feel good, period! And muscle burns fat! The more muscle you make, the more fat you will burn. (Women: Muscle does not make you look "big." Quite the opposite. Most of my female clients see their size go *down* as their muscle mass goes *up*!)

I tell people to throw away their scales. It is no measure of success. Haven't you noticed that even though two people are the same height and weight, one can look flabby while the other looks fabulous? The reason is that one stores fat while the other stores muscle. Since muscle weighs more than fat, it's possible for a lean person to look slimmer than a flabby person who weighs less. How we look and how we feel depends on our ratio of fat to lean mass: our *body composition*. Ideal body composition is 10 to 15 percent fat for men and 15 to 20 percent fat for women. Bodybuilders and superathletes with "supercut" bodies are likely to have single-digit ratios. The majority of Americans, however, are carrying at least twice as much fat as they should!

And here's the real shocker. Sometimes it shows, and sometimes it doesn't!

It's possible for someone to be thin on the outside and fat on the inside. There are millions of people, primarily women, who fall into this "thin/fat" category. To stay slim, they subsist on very low-calorie diets, at great personal cost. They walk around tired, hungry, and frustrated that they can't eat normal meals. If they depart even slightly from their draconian diets, they blow up like balloons. The reason is nutrient partitioning. Most of the nutrients they consume are parked as fat. The only way they can keep weight off is to consume too few nutrients. The cycle is vicious. Because they don't have enough muscle—in fact, on these low-calorie diets, they're *losing muscle*—they don't burn fat efficiently. Therefore, they can only maintain their figures by starving themselves. It only gets worse with time. They may look fine on the outside, but inside they are a complete metabolic and physiological mess. Yet, if these same people follow my program and improve their lean-mass-to-fat ratio, they can stop starving themselves, eat real food, and not only look good but feel—and be—well.

On my program you will achieve what dieters have only been able to dream about: *You will build muscle and give 100 percent of the bill to fat.*

Julie: Tale of a Thin/Fat Woman

Julie is 28, pretty, slim, and a regular at my gym. She used to be the classic thin/fat woman. She could only maintain her figure by not eating. For years she lived on salads, low-fat yogurt, and tiny morsels of chicken or fish. She measured out her life in calories, trying to eat as few as possible. In the mistaken belief that it would keep her thin, she often skipped meals. She was always hungry and perpetually tired, but would spend hours a week on the stair stepper. Her mood would rise or fall, depending on whether her weight was slightly up or down. Her sense of well-being was measured in ounces!

Julie was a "disaffected dieter," typical of young female dieters today. You wouldn't know it by looking at her, but Julie was locked in fat-storage mode. Although she was slender, she had very little muscle. Every time she ate real meals, with normal-size portions, her body billowed, storing nutrients as fat in places she didn't like.

When I first met Julie, she begged for a diet to "help keep me thin." She was shocked when I told her that her predicament was the direct result of her constant dieting! I explained that her problem wasn't that she was eating too much; rather, she was eating too little—especially of the foods that would keep her in fat-burning mode. She was very resistant to the notion of eating more, and it took some convincing to get her to eat enough to feel satisfied. I put her on the 6-Pack Prescription Meal Plan, which had her eating more food in one day than she was accustomed to eating in three. I told her to spend less time on the treadmill and more time in the weight room. Within a month she no longer needed convincing. To her surprise she looked sleeker and better toned. The best part, she conceded, was that now that her metabolism was working with her and not against her, her shape and weight were easy to maintain. Oh, and she's not hungry and tired anymore.

I urge people like Julie to stop counting calories because when it comes to body composition, calories play a secondary role to nutrient partitioning. Your body composition will vary depending on whether you are eating 2,000 calories a day of the right food versus 2,000 calories of the wrong food. By eating the right food, you will be trim and strong and feeling satisfied. By eating the wrong food, you will be fat, flabby and constantly hungry. If you don't believe me, I've got the studies—and the bodies—to prove it.

Julie has never stepped on a scale since and has never been happier. She doesn't need a scale to know that the 6-Pack Prescription is working, and neither will you. You'll know it because in short order your clothes will fit more comfortably. Then you will have to tighten your belt a littler tighter to hold your pants up. Save up! Soon you will find yourself shopping for smaller sizes.

My Journey from the Gym to the ICU

Throughout my career, I have had one foot in the intensive-care unit and one foot in the gym. The gym and the ICU may strike you as worlds apart, but in fact, what I learned in the ICU I applied in the gym, and what I learned in the gym I applied in the ICU.

As a teenager, I became fascinated with competitive weight lifting, a sport that requires tremendous strength and muscle. I trained hard and lived on a high-protein diet of eggs (lots of eggs) and several pounds of beef a day. By the time I was 18, I was 300 pounds of sheer muscle. I know what you're thinking, but I was no dumb jock! I graduated first in my high school class, and got myself admitted to Boston University with the goal of pursuing a career in medicine. After graduating from college, I enrolled in the Boston University School of Medicine. I did my postgraduate medical training at Harvard's Massachusetts General Hospital and was a Senior Fellow in Intensive Care Medicine at Stanford.

Given my background as a bodybuilder, you might have assumed that I would have chosen a specialty in sports or rehabilitation medicine, but as a medical student and a doctor I became very intrigued with the problem of wasting syndrome in critically ill patients. At first glance, my choice of study may seem a bit odd, but in reality, wasting syndrome is all about muscle, or more accurately, the inability to make muscle and to keep muscle. Many severely injured or ill people do not die as a direct result of the injuries or specific diseases for which they seek treatment. Rather, they die of wasting syndrome, which is an extreme example of nutrient partitioning gone awry. Although they are fed a high-calorie diet intravenously, patients who are suffering from wasting syndrome are locked in a state of severe catabolism. Catabolism means that their nutritional traffic cop is basically off duty. Nutrients are not being parked. Nutrients and calories just flow through you. In order to stay alive, the body consumes its own muscle and lean tissue. The body cannibalizes itself. If proper metabolism is not restored, a catabolic or wasting patient will die of nutrient deprivation.

Although I was fascinated by the study of metabolism and nutrition, I discovered that nutrition is a gaping hole in the medical school curriculum. The courses just aren't there. I filled the gap with independent research and had the opportunity to study with some of the most renowned authorities on metabolic physiology at MIT and Harvard. I have since funded the establishment of the A. Scott Connelly Laboratory for Nutritional Sciences at the UCLA Center for Human Nutrition, so that tomorrow's doctors will be better informed.

Intensive Care for a Broken Metabolism

My study of wasting syndrome taught me that to fix a broken metabolism, you have to feed it the nutrients it needs, when it needs them. If you're not eating enough of the right nutrients and eating them often enough, your metabolism cannot work effectively. That special protein formula that I developed for patients who are seriously ill treats wasting syndrome by providing the nutrients required to rescue the metabolism and restore it to good working order.

My research also taught me that it is not just the chronically ill and seriously injured whose metabolisms are in dire need of rescue. Too many of us are sabotaging our metabolisms by failing to eat the right foods at the right times. As a result, we appear to be suffering from an odd version of wasting syndrome: We burn muscle to provide the nutrients necessary to keep our bodies running while storing the nutrients we *don't* need as fat. We are malnourished, our metabolisms are malfunctioning, and the effects are apparent in how we look, how we feel, and how we feel about how we look.

R_x: Protein

When I said *malnourished* earlier, I meant it. It may surprise you to learn that in this land of plenty, protein deficiency is rampant. In our modern diet, protein has been pushed to the side of the plate and supplanted by highly processed, refined foods, primarily starchy carbohydrates. On average, between 12 and 15 percent of our daily calories come from protein, and while that may be enough to enable us to survive, it is nowhere near enough to permit us to thrive. To escape fat-storage mode, you shouldn't starve yourself or restrict your diet beyond belief. Instead, you have to eat more protein, plain and simple.

If you want to shut down your metabolism and stay in fat-storage mode permanently, stay on the standard diet prescription—the high-carbohydrate, low-protein, low-fat, low-calorie diet. There is a reason why most dieters fail and not only gain back the weight they lost but actually gain back *more fat*. When you follow a high-carb, low-calorie diet, you may lose weight but you don't necessarily lose fat, and you also lose muscle. On the typical weight-loss diet, you will lose about 65 percent fat and 35 percent lean mass. When you go off the diet, which most people do because it's so unsatisfying, you gain the weight back primarily in the form of fat. Those new pounds consist of 80 percent fat and only 20 percent lean mass. Each time you go on and off your diet, you progressively chew up more muscle and make more fat.

This doesn't happen if you eat enough protein. I participated in a study at Texas Christian Women's University in which we put two groups of middle-aged obese women on a low-calorie diet and strength-training program. Although both groups consumed the same number of calories, one group ate more protein and fewer carbohydrates, and the other group ate more carbohydrates and less protein. Both groups of women lost substantial amounts of weight, but that was only half the story. The group on the low-protein diet lost the standard 65 percent fat, 35 percent lean mass that is the standard result of most low-calorie diets. *The women on the high-protein diet lost almost exclusively fat.* The additional protein turned on the metabolic fat-burning machinery while preserving muscle and lean mass. In other words, the cost of making muscle was billed to their fat cells! In addition, the women on the high protein diet enjoyed yet another advantage. While they were on the diet regimen, they experienced a significant increase in their metabolic rate, whereas the women on the low-protein regimen had a decrease in the metabolic rate. In other words, the group eating more protein burned more energy—that is, more calories—throughout the day than the group eating less protein.

Protein is the key metabolic currency of the body. Your body was designed to run on it. Protein molecules drive all the chemical reactions involved in the breakdown and absorption of food, including carbohydrates and fat. In other words, protein drives virtually all aspects of metabolism. Many studies, including some of my own, show that simply adding protein to your diet turns on your fat-burning/muscle-building switch—even if you make no other lifestyle changes. When I gave one group of bodybuilders extra protein along with their normal diet, they gained *two times* as much muscle mass as a second group of bodybuilders doing exactly the same workout and eating the same diet but without the extra protein. When you're stuck in fat-storage mode, you need a powerful protein boost to jump-start your metabolism back into fat-burning mode. In most cases, you cannot easily get enough protein from food alone to do the job. To fill the protein gap, in addition to increasing protein consumption through food, I recommend a daily high-potency protein powder. It is a simple, safe, efficient way to repair your metabolism and build a lean, shapely body.

Adding Protein Is More Important Than Cutting Carbs

This isn't the same all-protein, noncarbohydrate prescription you've heard before. I strongly disagree with diet gurus who contend that a high-protein diet will work only if you give up most carbohydrates, including good carbohydrates such as fruits and many vegetables. Those low-carbohydrate/high-protein diets are designed to create a biochemical condition within the body called ketosis, which promotes the formation of chemicals called ketones. Your body eliminates ketones by flushing them out through urine. Anyone who has ever been on a high-protein, virtually no-carbohydrate diet knows you spend a lot of time in the bathroom! The problem is, you may lose a lot of weight at first, but much of it is water weight. Over time, ketogenic diets can cause nasty side effects like bad breath, constipation, and sallow-looking skin and may even cause kidney damage. Moreover, their high fat content may put susceptible people at much greater risk for heart disease. And since very low-carbohydrate diets are so restrictive, they're difficult to stay on. They get very boring! Those who do persevere find that they are consuming less food because eating protein and little else is very unappealing. Try it for a few days and you'll see what I mean! Ultimately these diets become low-calorie diets, if not by design, then by default. And any low-calorie diet is going to wreak havoc on your metabolism.

There is another fundamental flaw with diets that are too low in carbohydrates. If you don't eat enough carbohydrates, you cannot utilize protein properly. As a result, a diet too low in carbohydrates can actually prevent you from building muscle and staying lean. The very diet you think is helping you may be hindering your progress! Just like Julie, people on these diets must watch every morsel that goes into their mouths lest they put the weight back on again.

The 6-Pack Prescription is not a ketogenic diet: You can eat virtually unlimited amounts of good carbohydrates, like most fruits and vegetables, and don't even have to give up all starchy carbohydrates such as bread, potatoes, and pasta. In fact, you can eat up to *ten times* the amount of carbohydrates on my meal plan as you can on the well-known ketogenic diets, yet you will become a champion fat burner. Why? These diet doctors have it all backwards. They stress cutting out carbohydrates: I stress adding protein. And I add a lot more protein than they do, but I do it safely.

First, unlike foods in other high-protein diets, the protein foods that I recommend are low in saturated fat. Thus, they are good for the heart. As a physician, I think that pushing high-fat sources of protein is completely irresponsible. I've heard the argument that these diet doctors use—that a high-fat diet doesn't cause heart disease. I don't buy it. I've spent too many years in the ICU treating heart patients to be cavalier about the risk of heart disease. An unknown percentage of people will get atherosclerosis (clogged arteries) from a high-fat diet, and *we don't know who they are until it happens.* That's not a risk I'm willing to take with my life, and I don't think you should be either. That's why the 6-Pack Prescription Meal Plan stays well within reasonable fat guidelines.

Second, the 6-Pack Prescription Meal Plan is kind to your body. I'm not trying to get you to slim down by intentionally creating an unhealthy imbalance in your body. Instead, the 6-Pack Prescription Meal Plan works so well because it *restores* balance. Because you are eating enough carbohydrates, you are never in ketosis and never suffer its nasty side effects. Of course, I tell you to cut out the junk carbohydrates while giving advice on which carbohydrates are best, but there's never a day when you cannot have bread, pasta, or potatoes. And there's never a day when you're going to feel deprived.

R$_x$: Fiber

Fiber is another important nutrient that has all but vanished from our food supply. Chances are, you are not getting enough fiber, and because of that, your metabolism is suffering. Most Americans eat between 10 and 15 grams of fiber a day. You may say, "So what. I just read about a study that showed that eating fiber doesn't prevent colon cancer. Why should I eat fiber?" The answer is simple: *Fiber burns fat. And protein and fiber together are the most powerful fat-burning food combination there is.*

Good carbohydrates such as fruits and vegetables are a great source of fiber, but most of us don't eat enough of them. (Many of us don't eat any.) I don't want to sound like your mom. So I'll put it this way: Eat your fruits and vegetables if you want to look better naked. If you just can't stand to eat enough fruits and vegetables to get your fiber, there are a few shortcuts that I'll tell you about later.

R~x~: No Fructose

If you want to look better naked, and if you want to live better longer, reduce your intake of fructose! Fructose is the primary sweetener used in processed foods, and it's also used as a stabilizing agent in frozen food to prevent freezer burn.

Fructose is the Stealth bomber of sweeteners. It gets into your cells by coming in below the radar. It doesn't cause a sudden rise in blood sugar like table sugar, which is why it's considered safe enough for diabetics. The reality is, fructose is far more insidious than real sugar—not just for diabetics, but for everyone. Eating fructose is like taking a giant fat pill! Scientists have discovered that fructose has an immediate and dangerous effect on metabolism. It sets your metabolism in fat-storage mode and keeps it there.

Fructose is ubiquitous throughout the food supply. You will find it listed on food labels as "high-fructose corn syrup" or "natural fruit sweeteners." If you walk through the aisles of a supermarket and read the labels, you're in for a shock. High-fructose corn syrup is just about everywhere—in cereals, breakfast bars, cookies, sweetened beverages, salad dressings, energy bars, ice cream, candy bars, marinades, frozen entrées, desserts, and even many alleged health foods. As much as 16 percent of our daily calories come from fructose. Kids who live on sugary, processed foods consume even more than that. At one time, fructose was touted as healthier for us than other forms of sugar. We now know that it's not, and as I explain in Chapter 3, "The 'F' Word in Nutrition," to the contrary, it's a lot worse for us.

The 6-Pack Prescription

The 6-Pack Prescription is a nutrition and fitness program consisting of four different six-week cycles, each with a different strategy and goal:

Cycle 1: "6 Weeks to Strength"

Cycle 2: "6 Weeks to Sculpt"

Cycle 3: "6 Weeks to Burn Fat"

Cycle 4: "6 Weeks to Maintenance and Endurance."

My 6-Pack Prescription Meal Plan and weight-training method work synergistically to produce results quickly, safely, and extraordinarily effectively. Some of you may wonder: "Do I have to do both to get great results?" I understand that some of you may be intimidated by the mere thought of lifting weights but may be willing to do the meal plan. Some of you may love lifting weights but may not want to follow the meal plan. As far as I'm concerned, nutrition is the cornerstone of my program. If you want to change your body, first and foremost you need to change how you eat. As good as weight training may be, if you don't eat correctly, you can easily negate all the good things you are doing for yourself at the gym. Even if you never step into a gym, you can achieve great results by eating properly. But your results will be even more astounding if you follow my 6-Pack Prescription WorkOut method and Meal Plan together. If you choose only to start with either the meal plan or the workout program, my hope is that once you see the great result you will get with one part of the program, you will be eager to start the other.

The 6-Pack Prescription Meal Plan

The 6-Pack Prescription Meal Plan is designed to liberate you from fat-storage mode. It does it by putting protein and fiber back into your meals and by gradually decreasing the amount of starchy carbohydrates that you consume. You will shift your eating patterns every six weeks to achieve the goals of each cycle. At no point will you feel hungry, deprived, or bored with your diet. You will probably feel as if I'm asking you to eat *too much, too often*. As I often tell my clients, the only way you can "cheat" on my program is by not eating enough food.

I will show you how to monitor your daily consumption of three nutrients: protein, fiber, and carbohydrates (only the starches). The daily protein requirement per person varies according to your weight and the cycle you are in. In your 6-Pack Prescription Meal Planner, you'll find all the charts that make this a no-brainer.

When it comes to following a meal plan, simplicity rules! With rare exceptions, most people eat the same twelve to fifteen foods over and over again, day in and day out. Of course, we're often eating the wrong foods. The 6-Pack Prescription makes it easy for you to switch to twelve to fifteen of the right foods. To make life simple, I've divided the world of food into three ratings, Green, Yellow, and Red. Green is the best: These foods are all but unlimited. Yellow signals caution: These are the foods that you should keep careful track of. Red means stop: Avoid these foods whenever possible. The charts on pages 164–175 help make this simple to follow. As you progress through the cycles, you will gradually increase your consumption of green proteins and decrease your consumption of yellow carbohydrates. Your 6-Pack Prescription Meal Planner will help you keep track of what and when you are eating, and sample menus for each can be of great help.

To make life especially easy, I've put all the food plan charts, planners, and menus into a book-within-a-book located in Chapter 5.

R$_x$: Put Muscle Back in Your Metabolism

Why weight training?

Because weight lifting is the only form of exercise that can build muscle and lean mass. Weight lifting changes your body composition from fat to lean quickly and effectively. Remember, muscle is the engine that runs your metabolism. Muscle gets you into fat-burning mode and keeps you there. Muscle burns more fat than other tissue, even when your body is at rest (which is 70 percent of the time). The more muscle you have, the more fat you burn, the faster you burn it, and the more you can eat and still stay lean. The 6-Pack Prescription will teach you how to turn your muscle into a world-class fat burner.

There is a common misconception among women that weight training will give them big, bulging muscles everywhere, while aerobics will slim them down in the right places. Not so! There is nothing that aerobics can do for your body that weight training can't do faster and better. Aerobics does not build muscle. Aerobic exercise turns up fat burning only during the time that you are exercising. Step off the stair stepper or the treadmill and your fat-burning ability plummets. In contrast, weight training turns up fat burning not only while you are exercising, but for days afterward. Even when you leave the gym, even when you are completely sedentary, you are still burning fat at a higher rate. Aerobics will not keep you from getting fat. In fact, under certain conditions, aerobics will slow your metabolism down to a crawl, especially if you are on a very low-calorie diet. In contrast, my weight-training program gives your body definition but no bulges. The result is an attractive, well-toned body. Even with your bigger muscles, you'll probably wear a smaller size. And this goes for men as well as women. If you don't believe me, look at our exercise model in Chapter 7. She went from a size 6 to a size 2 by following my workout prescriptions. (By the way, she's eating 1,000 calories a day more than when she was a size 6!)

The 6-Pack Prescription Workout

My weight-training system is extraordinarily effective, yet simple enough for beginners. If you've been spending a lot of time working out with no discernible benefits, I urge you to give my method a try. If *exercise* is a foreign word to you, give it a shot. No huge time commitment is required. The question is not how much time you spend working out, but how you spend it.

The basic weight-training program consists of twenty weight-training exercises divided into four separate workout sessions, each to be performed once a week. Each session should take under an hour. In other words, you'll spend less than one hour a day, four days a week in the gym. You can track your progress on the 6-Pack Prescription Workout Planner included in Chapter 7.

Each exercise is illustrated with easy-to-follow directions and advice to accommodate the needs of both beginners and more advanced weight lifters.

- Cycle 1, "6 Weeks to Strength," will strengthen your muscle fibers to build the foundation you will need for cycles 2 and 3.

- Cycle 2, "6 Weeks to Sculpt," will give you better muscle definition, emphasizing the replacement of fat stores with muscle tissue.

- Cycle 3, "6 Weeks to Burn Fat," will help you use your newly acquired muscle to maximize your body's fat-burning abilities.

- Cycle 4, "6 Weeks to Maintenance and Endurance," will help you keep your new body trim and enhance your ability to perform well, both in sports and in your daily activities of living.

Nothing to Lose, Everything to Gain

Traditional weight-loss programs emphasize the word *loss*. I believe that this reflects a very negative, self-defeating approach that is doomed to failure. My program is not about loss: It's about gain. You're not losing a part of your body, you're building up your body in a constructive, healthy way. You're making the muscle to drive your metabolic machinery while handing over the bill to fat. You're not depriving yourself of food, as you do on most low-calorie diets; rather, you're eating real food all day long.

And best of all, you will see results. Within a few weeks of starting the 6-Pack Prescription, you will notice that your body is stronger and more toned, and you feel more energetic. By the time you complete the 6-Pack Prescription, you'll look great in your clothes . . . or without them.

Many of you may be eager to get started on the 6-Pack Prescription

How To Use This Book

Body Rx is divided into three sections:

- Part I, "Throw Out Your Scale," describes how the principles of the 6-Pack Prescription can change your body.

- Part II, "How to Get the Body You Want," details the four cycles of the fitness and nutrition program.

- Part III, "Dr. Connelly's Intensive Care for Special Situations," offers specific advice for women and older people.

program. If you are ready to begin, go directly to Part II. It will provide all the tools you need to transform your body. Go right ahead and start the program, but do come back and review the basics in parts I and III.

In my experience, the most motivated people are those who understand *why* they are doing what they are doing. Therefore, I urge you to read parts I and III.

2

The Metabolic Meltdown

Picture this:

A thousand years from now, a team of anthropologists uncovers the remains of a city in the midwestern United States. The scientists are mystified by a strange and disturbing discovery. Their analysis of skeletal remains, clothing styles, and home videos reveals that toward the end of the twentieth century, Americans of all ages and all economic categories grew fatter . . . and fatter . . . and fatter. In fact, by the turn of the century, these Americans were the fattest people on the planet! The anthropologists are stumped. What, they wonder, triggered such a radical and unhealthy shift in body composition in such a short period of time?

I can only speculate how future scientists will view our inability to deal with this public health crisis, but as a physician it frustrates me to no end. It's not that we don't recognize the problem. Experts agree that Americans are getting fatter, but you don't have to take the experts' word for it. Take a walk anyplace where crowds gather—an airport, a shopping mall, the beach, a public pool—and one fact will be startlingly apparent: One out of every two American adults is overweight. This is not just a problem that afflicts adults. Go to the park, a playground, or a video arcade and you will see that one out of four American kids is also too fat.

Prevalence of Overweight in American Adults

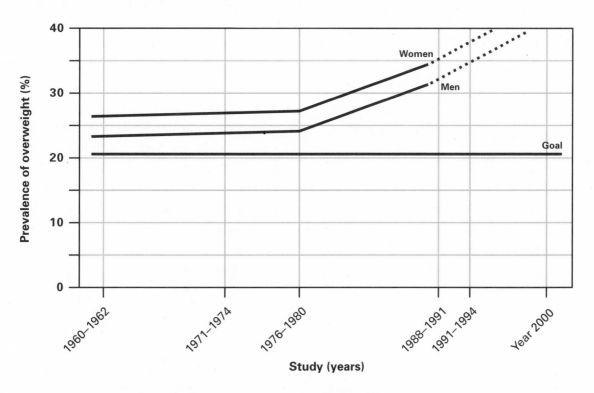

If you still doubt that obesity is a growing menace, take a look at the graph above. It is based on an ongoing study on obesity by the U.S. government, and it tracks changes in the number of overweight American adults from 1960 to the present. You will see that between 1960 and today there has been a dramatic increase in the number of overweight and obese Americans. Take a closer look at the graph and consider the following underlying data that went into creating it:

- Around the year 1980, there was a sudden and dramatic spike in obesity that continues unabated today.

- In the period 1991–1998, *there was a 60-percent increase in obesity among all adults.*

- In the period 1998–1999 (just one year!), there was a 6-percent increase in adult obesity.

- The incidence of childhood obesity has nearly doubled since 1960, most of the rise occurring in the past two decades.

This is not just a matter of looking good: It's a matter of being well. Obesity can kill you. Obesity greatly increases your risk of developing three serious metabolic disorders that occur so frequently that they are considered modern-day epidemics: Syndrome X, insulin resistance, and Type II or adult-onset diabetes. All these disorders involve insulin, the hormone that is essential for regulating the body's metabolism of sugar and starches as well as performing many other important jobs, including playing a critical role in the storage of fat and protein and the manufacture of cholesterol. The starchy, sugary foods typical of the modern diet cause a sharp rise in glucose (blood sugar) that triggers a spike in blood insulin levels. Too much insulin can cause trouble throughout the body.

Syndrome X is a recently discovered condition characterized by high levels of insulin, high blood pressure, and high levels of triglyceride, a type of fat found in the blood. Insulin resistance occurs when your cells respond to chronically high levels of insulin by becoming resistant to the hormone's effects. It is often a precursor to heart disease. In a similar condition, Type II or adult-onset diabetes, insulin works less efficiently, which increases the risk of heart disease, kidney damage, and even blindness. Once considered a disease of aging, Type II diabetes is, for the first time since we've been tracking the disorder, occurring much more frequently, rising 70 percent between 1990 and 1998 among people ages 30 to 39, and 40 percent among 40-to-49-year-olds. Another sign of the times: a sharp and unexpected increase in so-called adult-onset diabetes among children!

If this present trend continues, by the middle of this century close to three quarters of all American adults and one third of all children will be seriously overweight or heading that way. But in order to understand why the rate of obesity began to skyrocket after 1980—and, more importantly, what you can do to make sure you're not one of the obese— you need to understand the events leading up to this catastrophe.

Why Are We Fat?

No one doubts that obesity—with all its attendant health problems—is on the rise, but the question is: Why?

Some experts contend that we're getting fatter because we gorge on food and are so lazy that we don't burn off excess calories. They point accusatory fingers at supersized meals at fast-food restaurants, the popularity of video games, and endless hours spent watching television. Others theorize that the obesity epidemic is the result of a "fat gene."

I'm not going to take issue with the notion that chronic overeating and a failure to exercise can result in a fat and flabby body. In fact, I'm willing to concede that overconsumption—*especially overconsumption of the wrong foods*—plus an inactive lifestyle may explain some of the increase in obesity. And certainly there are some people who are genetically predisposed to being heavy. But none of these explanations can account for the marked increase in obesity that has occurred in the past two decades. If the "You're fat because you eat too much and do too little" theory is true, this would mean that sometime around 1980, all Americans, young and old, rich and poor, of all races, creeds and colors, suddenly resolved en masse to belly-up to the all-you-can-eat buffet while suddenly cutting out all exercise. Of course, that's ridiculous. If the "fat gene" theory is correct, then sometime around 1980 this gene abruptly got switched on. That doesn't make any sense either.

Studies show that Americans are not consuming significantly more calories than they used to and certainly not enough to warrant the sudden and inexplicable increase in obesity that has occurred since 1980. Nor are Americans more sedentary than they were twenty years ago. The percentage of physically active adults has remained fairly constant. When I was growing up in the 1960's, experts lamented the fact that American children were not as fit as children of prior generations because the family car had eliminated the need to walk to school! Today's children may be spending more time in front of video games and computers, but that's not the primary reason why kids are getting fatter.

If the obesity epidemic is not being caused by gluttony, laziness, or genetics, then what is to blame?

Obesity and poor body composition go hand in hand. People who are obese have too much body fat and too little muscle. Most of them were not born that way! The culprit is the modern diet. I—and a number of other researchers—believe that the continual rise in obesity that we have seen over the past fifty years and particularly in the past twenty is the result of radical changes in the Western diet that have occurred over these same periods. It's not that we're eating too much food, but that we're eating too much of the *wrong* food. The problem—and the solution—goes back to nutrient partitioning, the scientific concept that I introduced in Chapter 1. Nutrient partitioning, you will recall, is the metabolic traffic cop that directs nutrient traffic into either the fat parking lot or the lean-muscle parking lot. If you want a lean body, your metabolic traffic cop must direct more nutrients into the lean-muscle parking lot.

Foods and additives in our diet can "bribe" the metabolic traffic cop to direct nutrient traffic into either the lean-muscle parking lot or the fat parking lot. Positive partitioning agents are foods that do the former, promoting the formation of lean muscle and the burning of fat. Negative partitioning agents are foods and additives that do the latter, promoting the formation of fat. During the past half century, our food supply has become inundated with foods and additives that are negative partitioning agents. The past two decades have seen negative partitioning agents crowd out positive partitioning agents. And people are getting fatter with each passing year. Ironically, many of these foods are being marketed as "health" foods!

I believe that one food additive, high-fructose corn syrup, is a particularly potent negative partitioning agent. It has slowly and insidiously invaded our food supply, and I hold it largely responsible for the marked rise in obesity starting in the 1980's. I am so passionate about reducing the consumption of fructose that I devote the entire next chapter to this topic.

It's Nutrient Partitioning, Not Calories

I'm sure that some of you are thinking, *Wait a minute! What about calories? It's common knowledge that consuming too many calories will make you fat and that cutting back on calories will make you slim. According to the calorie theory, what you eat doesn't matter; how many calories of it you eat does.*

The common knowledge is wrong. No one has ever proven the calorie theory to be true. I'm not kidding! There isn't a single study that shows that if you feed people the same amount of excess calories, they will all gain the same amount of weight. Nor has anyone shown that if you deprive people of the same amount of calories, they will all lose the same amount of weight. It's not that simple. Human metabolism is far more complicated than that.

Calorie intake by itself does not determine body composition. The quality of the food you eat is even more important than the quantity. We all know people who eat relatively few calories and still have a high amount of body fat. Despite their miserly diets, these people actually look overweight. They may even believe some bankrupt theory about a slow metabolism or some such nonsense. We also know people who eat many more calories but who are muscular and trim. Why? Nutrient partitioning. *Nutrient partitioning is a phenomenon that puts calories in their place.* Unfortunately, the medical establishment in the U.S. has become so fixated on the calorie hypothesis that it automatically rejects any other theory, even when good science supports it.

European scientists are light-years ahead of us in the study and acceptance of nutrient partitioning. The earliest studies of nutrient partitioning were done on livestock, not humans. Fortunes rise and fall on the fat-to-lean content of animals raised for food, and this animal research produced groundbreaking findings clearly demonstrating that manipulation of the type of food fed to animals—not necessarily the number of calories—could create fatter or leaner animals. Later studies proved that the same principles work for humans. Nutrient partitioning is finally being recognized in the U.S. by physicians and scientists who do not want to repeat the failures of the past. Recently it has attracted the attention of bodybuilders, because victory in a bodybuilding competition can be as slim as a few ounces of fat.

It wasn't until I worked with patients who were suffering from wasting syndrome that I began to understand the power of nutrient partitioning. Wasting syndrome is a problem that often follows a severe injury or a severe illness. Even when wasting patients are fed an extraordinarily high-calorie diet—up to 5,000 calories daily—they do not necessarily gain weight. I saw many "overfed" wasting patients die from starvation. I didn't need much more proof that there were big holes in the calorie theory. There had to be another powerful force regulating metabolism. Years later I realized that the same force that was causing wasting disease could operate in reverse to make people fat.

Obesity and wasting are both nutrient-partitioning problems due to a metabolic breakdown. In the case of obesity, the metabolic traffic cops are so overwhelmed by a flood of negative partitioning agents that they divert too many nutrients to the fat parking lot and not enough to the lean-muscle parking lot. Thus, there's too much body fat and too little muscle. In the case of wasting, the metabolic police are so overwhelmed by the enormous demands imposed by illness that there is a complete derangement in metabolism. Starved for the right nutrients, the body begins to feed on itself.

In wasting syndrome, nutrients from food are not stored: They are burned for fuel. Despite a high calorie intake, the body is starved for more nutrients and will begin to devour its own tissues. Muscle is the first to go. Why? Muscle is the primary source of amino acids, the building blocks of protein, which are critical for the normal function of many systems, including the immune system and the brain. When you're wasting, your body rapidly depletes its stores of amino acids, which is why you quickly lose muscle tone and strength. From my own experience as a bodybuilder, I knew that the more protein I ate, the more muscle I made. During those rare times when I stopped following my high-protein regimen, I lost ground. I realized that simply inundating the body with calories wasn't going to stop wasting. In order to reverse wasting, you have to give the body the right balance of amino acids so that it will no longer deplete its own muscle. That's precisely why my protein formula worked, whereas the standard high-calorie diet did not. Once the metabolic police were given the right nutrients to meet the body's needs, they were able to restore normal metabolic traffic, and the wasting syndrome stopped. Paradoxically, the same approach works for obesity, but for different reasons. If you provide the metabolic police with the right nutrients, you will correct the metabolic glitch that is forcing the body to sock away fat and not make muscle. Just as adding calories will not cure wasting, simply taking away calories will not cure obesity.

The "3,500 Calories = 1 Pound of Fat" Myth

Let me give you some examples of nutrient partitioning in action that also demonstrate why the calorie theory is at best only part of the story. In a groundbreaking study conducted at a major Canadian university, twelve sets of male twins were overfed 1,000 calories a day for 84 days, a total of 84,000 excess calories per twin. If, as is commonly believed, 3,500 extra calories is equal to one pound of fat, then each man should have gained 24 pounds of fat over the course of the experiment, right? Wrong! That's not what happened. Some men gained as few as 9½ pounds while others gained as many as 29 pounds. Moreover, even though lean mass and muscle weigh more than fat, the men who put on the least weight were those who gained primarily lean mass and muscle, not fat. Why? Because of nutrient partitioning.

The men in the study who put on the most weight were governed by traffic cops that tended to divert nutrients toward the fat parking lot. Those who gained primarily lean mass and muscle were governed by traffic cops that tended to divert nutrients to the lean-muscle parking lot. Although there was a wide variation in weight gain between groups of twins, individual twin pairs showed a similar tendency to be either fat or lean. The twins in each set had a similar tendency to be either fat storers or fat burners. Their metabolic traffic cops walked the same beat.

This study also confirms the role of genetics in determining body type. A lucky few may eat all they want and still stay slim and lean. Like the twins in the study who gained the least amount of weight, these blessed individuals are also more likely to gain muscle and lean mass and burn fat. Most of us, however, are not that lucky. As noted in Chapter 1, most people are genetically programmed to be fat storers. Nevertheless, this doesn't mean that we have to throw in the towel and accept a less than desirable body composition. It does mean, however, that we have to be more careful about what we eat, and in particular, choose foods that help us overcome our genetic disadvantage.

Nutrient Partitioning in Action

Kids are born with a growth and development program that gives them a natural tendency to be lean, despite what they eat (which is why it's so shocking that children today are getting fatter and fatter!). Children and teenagers are awash in hormones and growth factors that encourage their bodies to park protein in lean mass and to burn fat. However, once we mature, we lose the hormonal advantages of youth and become more vulnerable to the effects of negative partitioning agents.

Over time, a diet rich in negative partitioning agents will take a serious toll. If you want to see a fast-forward version of the effects of negative partitioning, consider one side effect of the prescription drug prednisone. Prednisone is prescribed to treat pain and inflammation associated with conditions such as rheumatoid arthritis, lupus, and asthma. Anyone who has ever taken prednisone knows that one nasty side effect is that one gets fat very quickly. In fact, some people who take prednisone are so upset by the weight gain that they stop eating. Yet, they continue to put on weight. Prednisone is a powerful negative partitioning agent. Regardless of what you eat, prednisone promotes the burning of muscle for fuel, which rapidly consumes lean mass. If you use prednisone too long or too often, you will become weak and flabby, no matter how little you eat.

The good news about nutrient partitioning is that it is a phenomenon that we can control. Everything that I recommend in this book, including my 6-Pack Prescription Meal Plan, my workout regimen, and supplements, is designed to put you and keep you in positive-partitioning/fat-burning mode. Of all of these tools, however, I believe that nutrition is the most powerful. The right food can keep you in lean-mass/muscle-building mode. The wrong food can turn you into a relentless fat storer. Unfortunately, the modern diet is skewed in the wrong direction.

Lessons from the Past

You may be surprised to learn that many scientists believe that when it comes to nutrition, our paleolithic ancestors (whom we call "cavemen") were not so backward; in fact, they were way ahead of us. Dating back around 40,000 years ago, cavemen were hunter-gatherers. Their metabolic machinery was designed to handle what they could kill or find growing wild. Guess what? *Their* metabolic machinery is *our* metabolic machinery. Only the food supply has changed.

The two most striking differences between our diet and the hunter-gatherer diet are protein and starchy carbohydrate intake. Our ancestors ate two to three times the amount of protein that we eat, but the sources of protein that they ate—wild animals, game, fish—were much leaner than the hormone-fattened cattle and poultry brought to market today. Our ancestors consumed about the same amount of carbohydrates as we do today, but they did not consume the same kinds of carbohydrates that we do. They did not eat starchy breads, potatoes, pastries, and junk food, all of which can send glucose levels into the stratosphere. They ate fresh, raw vegetables, edible grasses (such as flax), raw nuts, and an occasional piece of fruit when it was in season. Due to their fruit and vegetable intake, our ancestors ate 100 to 150 grams of dietary fiber daily, which is eight to ten times more than the amount we eat today. Their diet also contained more good fats, such as omega-3 fatty acids (found in fish and plants), and fewer bad fats, such as the saturated fats (found in dairy and beef), than the modern diet.

Cavemen didn't need to take vitamin pills. The food they ate was packed with many more vitamins and minerals than the processed food we eat today. Scientists estimate that our ancestors' daily intake of vitamins and minerals was ten times higher than ours, primarily because the food was fresh and unprocessed.

How did our cavemen ancestors fare? Remarkably well. Anthropologists say that Stone Age men and women were taller and bigger-boned than modern humans. The average life span of cavemen was shorter than ours, but that was due to the dangerous times in which they lived, not chronic illness. Cavemen died because of famine or infection, or at the hands of their enemies. They did not suffer from two great modern-day killers, heart disease and diabetes, which are robbing people of their lives today. Moreover, despite the fact that they consumed a generous amount of calories—perhaps 3,000 calories daily—they were not fat. It's true that they were more physically active than we are today. However, I don't believe that exercise is the only reason that they stayed lean and muscular. The reason is that their diet was packed with positive partitioning agents—protein and fiber—foods that ran their metabolism like a well-oiled, fat-burning machine.

We continued to eat like cavemen until about 10,000 years ago. That's when we discovered how to plant seeds and grow crops. As we moved from a hunter-gatherer society to an agricultural society, breads, grains, and starches displaced protein and high-fiber grasses and vegetables as dietary staples. Breads, grains, and root vegetables (such as potatoes) prevailed because they were filling and tasty and because it was easier to grow these foods and store them than to track down sources of protein every day. But even thousands of years ago, the price of convenience foods was high. Within a few generations people lost a few inches of height, their bones began became thinner, their bodies became fatter, and for the first time they began to show signs of dental cavities and metabolic diseases such as heart disease and diabetes. These changes began to occur immediately, but only recently have obesity and metabolic diseases reached epidemic proportions. In the past fifty years we have managed to do more damage to our bodies than we have done over the past 100 centuries!

From Bad to Worse

The pace of damage has accelerated because of the most recent, dramatic changes in our food supply. Even after our ancestors became farmers, they still managed to produce and consume foods that contained a fair amount of fiber and other nutrients. Today we strip foods of fiber and nutrients in order to extend shelf life and make shipping easier. Our ancestors did not eat junk food, nor did they eat sweets, except on special occasions. Today we consume these foods in abundance and wash them down with gallons of soda. Our ancestors' diet kept their metabolism running smoothly. Today's low-protein, high-carbohydrate, highly processed diet short-circuits our metabolic machinery.

In order to produce the energy that runs our body, our metabolic machinery burns glucose. So, you think, the more sugar, the better: I'm giving my body the fuel it craves. But our bodies did not evolve in a high-sugar environment. A little bit of glucose goes a long way. Too much glucose clogs up the metabolic machinery.

If we don't overwhelm the body with glucose-producing foods, the body turns to other fuel sources. One is fatty acids released by our fat cells. In addition, the body burns short-chain fatty acids made from fiber fermented in your intestinal tract. Notably, the burning of fatty acids from fiber stimulates the release of even more fat from fat cells, causing your rate of fat burning to snowball dramatically. This is the power of fiber, and that's why I want you to eat so much of it.

So far, so good. But if you gorge on high-glucose-producing starchy carbohydrates (such as cereals, processed grains, and snack foods) and don't feed it enough fiber and protein, your metabolic machinery will be swamped with glucose. Starchy carbohydrates actively inhibit the burning of our stored fat for energy. Our bodies will utilize the glucose as fuel instead of burning fat. It's easier. And remember one of the key rules of nutrient partitioning: What doesn't get burned gets stored. Some of the carbohydrates that are not converted into glucose will be stored as glycogen in muscle cells, but muscle cells can store only small amounts. The excess carbohydrates will be stored as fat, and there is virtually no limit to the amount of fat we can sock away. To make matters worse, you are not burning any fat as fuel either. You compound the problem when you don't eat enough protein. Without adequate protein intake, the body begins to break down muscle, which makes you even fatter.

When you take protein out of your diet and replace it with foods that discourage fat burning, you are setting yourself up for a metabolic disaster. When you add protein to your diet, you will get leaner. The reason is what I call "the protein paradox."

According to the protein paradox, the more protein you eat, the more fat your burn. When you replace protein with high-glucose-producing foods, the tidal wave of glucose also produces a constant spike in blood insulin levels, which can lead to Syndrome X, insulin resistance, and Type II diabetes. You can see the same phenomenon occur in contemporary times whenever a primitive culture, living on a hunter-gatherer diet, suddenly comes in contact with the modern food supply. Within twenty years of the introduction of refined flour and sugar, you see a sudden spike in high blood pressure, insulin resistance, and heart disease.

Your Real Protein Requirements

When I think about our modern diet, I can't help but conclude that its main ingredients are a deadly combination of ignorance, politics, and the pursuit of convenience. The most important consideration—what our metabolism requires to function properly—just doesn't enter into the equation.

Consider the Food Guide Pyramid that was established by the USDA in 1992 to show Americans what to eat. What it really showed Americans was how to get fatter faster. The Food Guide Pyramid recommends 6 to 11 servings of glucose-producing starchy carbohydrates (like bread, pasta, and potatoes) and 2 to 3 servings of protein (like meat, eggs, and poultry) every day. Follow that recommendation and you will get fat.

The government's daily value (DV) for protein guidelines recommend about 50 grams of protein daily for women and 60 grams daily for men. This is not a lot of protein. Yet, many people, especially women, do not consume even this small amount of protein daily. As a result, they get fat.

Why is the DV for protein so low? The DV is not based on optimal intake to keep the body running well; rather, it is based on the minimal amount of a nutrient required to prevent illness. You are probably familiar with the DV for vitamins and minerals. For example, the DV for vitamin C is 60 mg daily. That is the amount needed to prevent a vitamin C–deficiency disease, such as scurvy. Yet, numerous studies have shown that in order to prevent heart disease and keep the immune system well functioning, humans need a minimum of 200 mg of vitamin C daily, and probably more than that. Our cavemen ancestors ate close to 1,000 mg in their food. Although the experts have stubbornly refused to revise the DV, millions of knowledgeable Americans take vitamin C supplements. When it comes to protein, the DV is based on what's required to keep you from getting sick, not on what's required to keep your body strong and healthy. That's why my 6-Pack Prescription Meal Plan recommends that you eat substantially more protein than the DV allowance.

Consuming enough protein is important for body composition because you can't make or maintain muscle without amino acids. Amino acids are stored primarily in muscle cells. If you don't get enough amino acids in your diet, your body is going to rob them from your muscle cells. This means that there won't be enough amino acids on hand to make new muscle cells or repair old muscle cells. The result is that you become fat and flabby. This is precisely what happens as we age. Once we stop growing, the primary job of our bodies is to maintain and repair our existing muscle mass. If your body does not get enough amino acids, it can't do its job.

The loss of muscle creates a vicious cycle in which you keep gaining fat while losing more muscle. Muscle is much more metabolically active than fat, which means it burns up more energy. Even better, muscle likes to burn fat for energy. If you constantly lose muscle, you will also be losing your body's natural fat-burning machinery, which helps keep you slim. The inevitable result is a weaker, flabbier body.

Have you noticed that we humans are the only large mammals on earth that progressively lose muscle and gain fat with each passing year? And that we lose strength and get frail in our later decades? This was not always the case. Our paleolithic ancestors were not only bigger and stronger than we are, but they didn't suffer the same kind of muscle wasting as they aged. Why? The generous amount of protein in their diet gave them enough amino acids to run their bodies and maintain their muscle tone. After we reach our full growth and development in our late teens and early twenties, we switch out of growth mode and into maintenance mode. As our systems wear out and break down, our cells need enough amino acids not only to keep things running but to do necessary repairs. If we are continually draining our supply of amino acids, this important work can't be done. I believe that much of the wasting and frailty so common in old age today can be virtually eliminated by simply increasing protein intake. (See Chapter 10, "It's Never Too Late.")

The Low-Calorie, High-Carbohydrate Folly

For the past twenty-five years, the standard prescription for weight loss has been a low-calorie diet. The most popular of these diets is the high-carbohydrate, low-fat diet. The same dietary strategy is also recommended for people who want to prevent heart disease. And because protein typically comes from higher-fat foods (like beef, eggs, and dairy), as fat is cut from the diet, so is protein. For years I've contended that this type of diet can have a harmful effect on body composition, leaving one fatter and flabbier than before. I'm not suggesting that eating all the fat you want is okay. It's not. A diet high in saturated fat can increase the risk of heart disease in some people. But the solution is not to replace fat with refined carbohydrates, which can be equally damaging by overloading the body with glucose. Recent studies suggest that the high-carbohydrate, low-fat diet is precisely the wrong mix of nutrients for our metabolism. The flood of glucose and the dearth of protein creates a nutrient-partitioning problem that rapidly shifts us into fat-storage mode.

If you follow a very strict low-calorie diet, you will probably lose some weight. You may even lose a lot of weight. But you will not be substantially leaner. Any low-calorie diet will have a disastrous effect on your metabolism. Chances are, you will end up a smaller version of your fat self. If you started on your diet at 25 percent body fat, you could end up with the same fat to lean-mass ratio. I don't think that is a good result. Without increasing muscle, it will be excruciatingly difficult to stay slim. You will find—perhaps you have already found—that you maintain your "thin-fat" body only by starving yourself. If you do begin to eat normally, you will not only put on more weight, but the weight that you put on will be in the form of fat. Indeed, the weight you put on will be much fattier than the weight you took off!

I want to make one thing clear: If you've failed at these diets, it's not your fault. *It's the fault of the diets.* The combination of low-protein, high-glucose-producing foods stacked the deck against you. There was no way that you could have succeeded.

Studies conducted at some of the nation's leading medical centers cast doubt on whether the high-carbohydrate, low-fat approach is either the best prevention against heart disease or the solution for obesity. In fact, there is compelling evidence that eating a high-carbohydrate, low-fat diet may actually *increase* your risk factors for heart disease and other deadly diseases. Why? Because these diets increase your production of fat! And the more fat your body makes, the worse off your body composition.

- The Dietary Alternatives Study conducted by researchers at Northwestern Lipid Research Center and the Department of Psychiatry and Behavioral Sciences, University of Washington School of Medicine, Seattle, investigated the effects of different levels of dietary fat intake on blood lipid levels in 531 male Boeing employees. All the participants had been previously diagnosed with either high cholesterol or high cholesterol and high triglyceride levels. The participants were divided into four groups and each group was fed a diet containing a different amount of saturated and unsaturated fat. The researchers found that the men who were on the most fat-restricted diets had a 20-to-40-percent increase in levels of plasma triglyceride (a blood fat), placing them at greater risk of insulin resistance and Syndrome X, which actually increases their risk of obesity.

- A groundbreaking study conducted at Rockefeller University in New York raises even more serious questions about low-fat, high-carbohydrate diets. The study, which included both lean and obese people, compared effects of a very low-fat (10 percent of daily calories), high-carbohydrate diet enriched with simple sugars with effects of a 30-percent-fat diet. The low-fat, high-carbohydrate diet not only raised blood triglyceride levels 30 to 50 percent higher than the 30-percent-fat diet, but did something even worse. It stimulated the production of new fatty acids. In other words, it made people fatter! This negative result did not just occur in subjects who were fat to begin with, or who were particularly carbohydrate-sensitive. It also occurred in subjects who were lean. In other words, whether you are fat or thin, a low-fat, high-carbohydrate diet can actually make your body produce more fat. I guarantee that if you stay on this diet long enough, you will get fat, whether or not you started out that way.

The low-fat, high-carbohydrate diets used in these studies are not unlike the diets followed by millions of Americans trying to stay slim and healthy. Supermarket shelves are packed with foods that are low in fat and high in refined carbohydrates and sugar. Because they are low-fat, many of these products are marketed as wholesome and healthy and as a better alternative to full-fat products. Even more damaging is the replacement of fat in processed food with a new ingredient, high-fructose corn syrup—one of the major contributors to the metabolic meltdown.

The "F" Word in Nutrition (It's Not Fat!)

If you were to go into your kitchen and start reading food labels with an eye toward finding the single most common ingredient in all processed or prepared foods, I have an idea what you'd find: *high-fructose corn syrup* (fructose for short). Fructose, a particular kind of sugar, is present in a wide assortment of processed foods, including baked goods, soups, snack foods, soda, condiments, frozen entrées, breakfast cereals, and candy bars. Fructose was originally developed as a low-cost alternative to sucrose, or what we call table sugar. However, today fructose is not only used as a sweetener. It has become a multipurpose food additive, and in many products it is more than just an additive: It is a major ingredient. You will find, for example, that fructose is the second listed—and thus the second largest—ingredient in many brands of tomato soup, ketchup, marinades, energy bars, and soda. You will find it in bread, frozen pizza, cereal, cookies, and canned fruit. Don't take my word for it. Look in your cupboard and refrigerator, and you will see for yourself that fructose is ubiquitous.

According to conservative estimates, in the thirty-odd years since fructose was introduced, fructose consumption in the U.S. has increased ten- to twentyfold. It has replaced added sugar in about half of all processed food products. This increase has come as our craving for low-fat or no-fat foods has skyrocketed. One of the reasons food manufacturers add fructose to foods that are low-fat or fat-free is that, in addition to acting as a sweetening agent, it improves the "mouth feel" of processed foods. Fructose also extends the shelf life of frozen food. As fructose is less expensive than other sweeteners and preservatives, manufacturers are using it in a growing number of products, including many that are marketed as health foods. Consumption of fructose is rising, not because we're eating more food, but because we're eating more food to which fructose has been added.

Should we care that the food supply is being saturated with high-fructose corn syrup? Is it really worse than any of the other sweeteners and additives injected into the modern food supply?

The answer to both questions is yes. There is compelling scientific evidence demonstrating that fructose, more than any other single ingredient, is responsible for the obesity epidemic sweeping the U.S. I blame overconsumption of fructose for the unprecedented rise in obesity among children and teenagers, many of whom consume an endless stream of soda, snacks, and other fructose-laden foods. Moreover, I believe that unless we take steps to reduce our intake of fructose, the obesity epidemic will continue to rage out of control.

Ironically, fructose has been promoted as being healthier than table sugar, when research shows it to be much worse. I am not suggesting that table sugar is a health food. It's not. In Chapter 2, I explained how starchy, sugary foods are precisely the wrong foods for our metabolism because they are negative nutrient-partitioning agents that promote the storage of fat. But as problematic as sugar is, fructose is worse.

I want to assure you that if you occasionally eat a food product containing fructose, you will not be endangering your health. In fact, I've used fructose in small—actually minuscule—amounts in some of my own products. When used as an additive and not a primary ingredient (the way I believe that fructose was meant to be used), fructose is harmless. The problem is that fructose has invaded the food supply and is being consumed in quantities that I believe may be health-threatening. Let me explain why.

What Is Fructose?

Fructose, also known as levulose, or fruit sugar, is found in small amounts in fruits and to a lesser extent in vegetables and in higher concentrations in juice. It is the sweetest of the various kinds of sugars. High-fructose corn syrup, which is identical to the fructose found in nature, is a chemically altered version of corn syrup.

I'm not suggesting that you stop eating fruits because they contain fructose. Despite their sweet taste, when you eat fruits, you actually get a tiny amount of pure fructose along with other good stuff, like water, fiber, and beneficial phytochemicals (disease-fighting substances), vitamins, and minerals. When you eat a processed food product with fructose, you are getting a highly concentrated form of fructose minus all the beneficial ingredients found in fruits and vegetables.

Fructose and Your Health

When it was first introduced, high-fructose corn syrup was thought to be a healthier sweetener, because when fructose is metabolized it doesn't trigger as sharp a spike in insulin levels as table sugar does. Elevated insulin levels are linked to several serious health problems, including insulin resistance, Syndrome X, and Type II or adult-onset diabetes. You may already be familiar with the glycemic index (GI), which is a system for rating foods according to how they affect blood sugar and insulin levels. Foods with low GI ratings are considered to be healthier than those with high GI ratings, because they stimulate the release of less insulin. On the glycemic scale, table sugar rates a high 59. High-fructose corn syrup rates a low 20. Due to its low GI rating, fructose has been touted as a safe sugar for diabetics. However, there is substantial evidence that fructose poses a far more serious health threat than table sugar does. Indeed, scientists believe that the health risks associated with table sugar result from the fact that table sugar is 50 percent fructose!

In Chapter 1, I referred to fructose as the "Stealth bomber of sweeteners," because although it does not cause an immediate spike in glucose and insulin levels, there is a compelling body of scientific evidence, dating back to the 1960's, that shows the less immediate but long-term damaging effects of fructose. Dr. John Yudkin, M.D., chairman of the Department of Nutrition at London's Queen Elizabeth College, was one of the first researchers to call attention to the link between heart disease and sugar consumption. Dr. Yudkin discovered that a diet high in sucrose (table sugar) resulted in elevated blood levels of cholesterol, triglycerides, insulin, cortisol, and uric acid. So much for sucrose. What about fructose? When Dr. Yudkin performed the same experiment using pure fructose instead of sucrose, he found that fructose caused blood levels of cholesterol and triglycerides to soar nearly twice as high.

Back in the 1960's, Dr. Yudkin and other scientists who suggested that a high-sugar, high-carbohydrate diet was dangerous were dismissed as extremists and "health food types" or simply ignored. Organizations such as the American Medical Association and the American Heart Association continued to promote the virtues of a high-carbohydrate, low-fat diet, without cautioning against sugar consumption. Inexplicably, in 1986, when the U.S. Food and Drug Administration Sugars Task Force investigated the extraordinary increase in sugar consumption in the U.S., a panel of experts concluded that steadily rising sugar consumption did not pose a problem. These experts found no conclusive evidence that sugar consumption caused any adverse health effects other than cavities. I don't know what studies these experts were looking at, because even by the mid-1980's, study after study had documented that overconsumption of sugar in general, and fructose in particular, posed a significant health hazard. Today some of the world's most serious researchers are taking a second look at fructose and are not liking what they see:

- Dr. Judith Hallfrisch, a researcher at the National Institute on Aging, analyzed the major studies on fructose and its effect on health. Her findings were worrisome. "With regard to blood lipids, there is overwhelming evidence that fructose increases plasma triglycerides. Under some conditions, dietary fructose may cause increases in plasma cholesterol." In other words, fructose can increase the amount of fatty deposits in the blood, which in turn can increase the risk of developing insulin resistance, Syndrome X, adult-onset diabetes, and heart disease.

- Fructose can switch metabolism from fat burning to fat storage mode by promoting the formation of long-chain fatty acids, which are resistant to oxidation. Remember the rules of nutrient partitioning—what doesn't get oxidized (i.e., burned for fuel) gets stored in the body. Therefore, the more long-chain fatty acids you produce, the more fat you will have on your body.

- A particularly alarming study, conducted at the Children's Cardiovascular Health Center at Columbia-Presbyterian Medical Center, examined the diets of sixty-seven children between the ages of two and ten being treated for high cholesterol. All of the children were placed on a fat-restricted diet. On the basis of food diaries maintained by parents, the researcher found a link between the intake of simple carbohydrates (sugar) and low HDL (high-density lipoprotein), the good cholesterol, which helps prevent heart disease. The more fructose they ate, the lower their level of good cholesterol.

- Fructose can increase the amount of uric acid produced by the body, which may increase the risk of developing gout, a common form of arthritis.

- A high-sugar diet, particularly one laden with fructose, may actually make you look and feel old before your time. Both glucose and fructose can damage proteins in the body, resulting in the formation of what scientists call "advanced glycation end products" (or AGE products for short). AGE products not only cause noticeable damage, such as wrinkles and age spots, but in high amounts, AGE products can do internal harm to joints and vital organs, including the heart and eyes. Studies suggest that fructose is ten times more likely than sucrose or glucose to trigger the formation of AGE products.

- A study conducted by USDA scientists found that fructose may also increase the risk of osteoporosis, the degenerative bone disease that makes the elderly more vulnerable to breaks and fractures. Scientists believe that fructose may disrupt the normal balance among magnesium, calcium, and phosphorus, minerals that are essential for the construction and maintenance of bone, particularly in the context of a low-magnesium diet. They caution, "Further studies are warranted to see if a high-fructose diet with low dietary magnesium and marginal calcium leads to bone loss."

The studies that I refer to above are all short-term studies. Thus, they don't answer a very critical question: What are the long-term effects of eating a high-fructose diet? Clearly, there are some worrisome short-term effects, particularly for blood lipid levels and fat metabolism; yet, in the absence of long-term studies, we can only surmise about the long-term harm. We have no evidence that children are immune to the adverse metabolic effects identified in adults. We should be particularly concerned about the fact that the major consumers of fructose are the very young, who are exposed to this product at high doses early in life and for the longest terms. I believe that they are already paying a steep price in terms of their overall health and body composition.

Poisoning the Well

If one picture is worth a thousand words, then the chart on page 51 speaks volumes about the relationship of fructose to the current obesity epidemic. The chart tracks the increase in BMI, or body mass index (a measurement that compares a person's actual weight and height to ideal weight and height), against the introduction of new food products, such as baked goods, sweetened beverages, cereals, and snack foods. A BMI over 25 is considered overweight, and increases your risk of having a chronic illness that can shorten your life. If you look at the chart you will see that beginning in 1980, there was a sharp rise in the rate of obesity that continues unabated today. What is it that happened in 1980 that might have suddenly triggered the obesity epidemic? Did we all decide to gorge on cheesecake? The answer lies in the food supply. Think about the new food products brought to market over the past two decades. What do many of them have in common? Fructose. Fructose is skewing the national metabolism in the fat-storage direction. I liken fructose in the food supply to poison in the well: It affects the entire community. Consider this chart in light of the fact that the rate of obesity is rising among all age, economic, and societal groups. However, kids are being hit the hardest. Why? In a word, fructose.

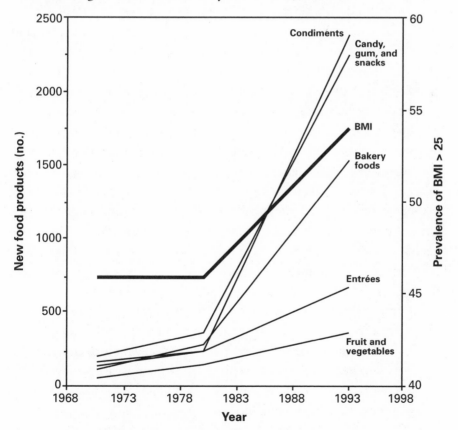

Reprinted with permission from the *American Journal of Clinical Nutrition*. © Am J Clin Nutr. American Society for Clinical Nutrition.

The Littlest Victims

Recently, while having breakfast in a coffee shop, I observed at the next table a young mother and her two small children. The mother was perusing *The Wall Street Journal* while sipping coffee. Her children were devouring a hearty breakfast consisting of a plate of waffles bathed in strawberry compote and whipped cream plus a giant-size chocolate-chip muffin, washed down by a large glass of apple juice.

What's wrong with this picture?

These kids were eating pure sugar with a fructose chaser with hardly a morsel of protein or fiber on the table. I can only assume that this obviously intelligent mother was utterly clueless to the fact that she was feeding her children a menu that would ensure them a lifetime of poor health.

Unfortunately, the scene that I just described is not an isolated incident. It is an accurate reflection of how kids eat in the U.S., both in and out their homes. Children and teenagers are the primary consumers of both sugar and fructose in the U.S. In fact, kids age 6 to 11 get 18 percent of their daily calories from added sugars, and teenagers get about 20 percent of their calories from added sugars.

The increase in obesity among children directly parallels the introduction of new food products, many of which did not exist before 1980, and many of which contain high-fructose corn syrup. As more and more processed food products were brought to market, and more and more manufacturers switched to high-fructose corn syrup, kids got fatter. Today, 24 percent of all children are so fat as to endanger their future health and well-being.

The problem is not just what children are eating. It's also what they're *not* eating. What they aren't eating is protein and fiber. In fact, food surveys show that kids age 12 to 19 typically do not consume even the paltry amount of protein that the government recommends.

Instead of foods that will help their bodies develop properly, kids are eating tons of sugar. Sugar overload begins during the earliest days of life. Many parents would be shocked to learn that many of the foods that they consider to be healthy and nutritious for their children are actually doing them harm. For example, 90 percent of all babies are fed fruit juice in their bottles before they reach the age of 1, and young children routinely drink juice daily. Most parents wouldn't dream of giving soda to their babies and young children; yet, in terms of sugar content, juice is not much better. It takes eight apples to make an 8-ounce glass of pure apple juice—that's a huge amount of fructose—and many kids drink more than one cup of juice a day. On top of all this juice, young kids are constantly eating highly sweetened cereals , crackers, cookies, and fruit yogurt treats (some of which are spiked with candy sprinkles). High-glucose-producing foods, such as candy and chips—once considered treats to be eaten rarely—have become dietary staples, and food manufacturers shamelessly market their products to young children. Within a short time after a new cartoon character is launched on television, sweetened cereals and fruit snacks based on that character appear on supermarket shelves. It's a good bet that these products are chock-full of fructose. (Moral: Don't take a cartoon character's endorsement of a product too seriously.) Moreover, there are hefty amounts of sugar and fructose lurking in foods that are not obvious snack foods, such as frozen pizza, waffles, bread, and breakfast bars.

Adolescents and teenagers binge on sugar all day long. They eat and drink it. The average teenage boy consumes 34 teaspoons of added sugar in his food daily, 44 percent of it from soda. He drinks 870 cans of soda a year! Teenage girls consume 24 teaspoons of sugar daily, 40 percent of it from soda. That's 800 cans of soda annually! Per capita consumption of soft drinks has increased almost 500 percent over the past fifty years. (Remember, most soda is basically nothing more than carbonated water, fructose, and a little flavoring.)

A recent study published in the British medical journal *Lancet* clearly demonstrated a link between obesity and the consumption of sweetened beverages, such as soda, iced tea, and fruit drinks. The study tracked the consumption of sweetened beverages by 548 public school children ages 11 and 12 from October 1995 to May 1997. It found that 25 percent of the children drank two or more extra cans a day of sweetened beverages at the outset of the study, and that 57 percent of the kids increased their intake of sugary drinks over the course of the study period. The researchers compared the daily consumption of sweetened beverages to the rate of obesity among the group, and the results were sobering. *Just one extra soft drink a day gave a child a 60-percent greater chance of becoming obese.* In fact, based on this study, each sugary drink consumed by a child daily contributed 0.18 points to their BMI. Remarkably, the researchers noted that the soft drink–obesity connection was independent of the food children ate, how much they exercised, and how much time they spent watching TV or playing video games. That means that regardless of what these kids ate or how much or how little exercise they got, drinking sweetened beverages increased their risk of obesity. The researchers noted: "Excessive body weight now constitutes the most common pediatric medical problem in the U.S.A. Although the cause of this apparent obesity epidemic is likely to be multifactorial, our findings suggest that sugar-sweetened drink consumption could be an important contributory factor." Although the study didn't mention fructose, it should have. It wasn't the water or the artificial coloring in the soft drinks that was making these kids fat. Fructose is the primary sweetener used in these popular beverages.

Kids don't even have to leave their schools to fill up on soda or sugar. Walk through any high school or junior high building and you will see vending machines dispensing soft drinks, candy, and chips. Ironically, I am told that the revenues generated from the sale of junk food are often used to support the school's sports teams.

Teenagers want to look good and feel good about their bodies and go to great lengths to achieve these goals. In fact, many teenagers resort to smoking or crash dieting in the belief that these unhealthy practices are the only way to maintain an attractive body. We need to teach kids at an early age that you don't have to sacrifice your health to look great. Having a great body is easy if you eat the right food.

What's missing is education, from the top on down. If parents don't know how to feed themselves—if they give their kids a steady stream of sugar, beginning in infancy—they can't expect kids to suddenly make intelligent choices on their own. Even people who believe that they are careful eaters are unaware of the high-fructose content in their food. Granted, we're not going to get kids to give up sugar entirely. But we can teach kids how to avoid hidden sources of sugar, and how to include some healthier foods in their daily diet. And there is no reason why manufacturers can't create healthier, fructose-free versions of foods that kids like to eat. Ultimately, it's up to parents to take food manufacturers to task for what I feel is nothing less than the poisoning of a generation.

4

Body R~x~: Nutrition

Good nutrition is the best tool we have to transform an unfit, flabby body into a trim, attractive body. It's even more powerful than exercise, you may be surprised to learn. The simple act of eating the right foods in the right amounts can produce a remarkable difference in your body composition, quickly and painlessly.

As I suspect you've gathered by now, good nutrition doesn't mean eating lousy food. I'm not talking about starving yourself, following a rigid diet, or eating things that you hate. I don't walk around hungry, and I don't eat stuff that I hate. I won't ask you to either. You'll still eat many of your favorite foods but you'll do it in a way that shows you understand that food can work with your metabolism, or against it.

The 6-Pack Prescription Meal Plan consists of four six-week cycles, each with a specific goal, and a six-week maintenance program, which you follow indefinitely. Over the eighteen-week meal plan, you will increase your consumption of foods that are natural fat burners, and decrease your consumption of foods that slow down fat burning. *The 6-Pack Prescription Meal Plan is not a low-calorie diet.* I don't want you to count calories; if you do, you could be sabotaging your efforts. Many of you will be eating more food, more often than you have in your lives; yet you will get leaner. As I said earlier, the only way you can fail on my program is by not eating enough fat-burning foods.

In this chapter, I will briefly review the science behind the 6-Pack Prescription strategy, so that you can understand more about the program and why it works. If you're ready to begin and don't want any further explanation, feel free to skip to Chapter 5, the 6-Pack Prescription Meal Plan, to get started. You can always read this section over as you begin to incorporate the program into your life.

Stop Starving Yourself!

Many of you have been told to stick to three meals a day and not eat in between or you'll get fat. Many of you walk around hungry in the mistaken belief that eating is what makes you fat. Wrong! Your metabolism works best when it is well fed throughout the day. The 6-Pack Prescription calls for six meals spread throughout the day, no more than three hours apart. Your food should be evenly divided among your six meals. I know that you've been taught to eat three meals a day, and in our culture we tend to eat our heavy meal at night. From the perspective of your metabolism, this is precisely the *wrong* way to eat. First, it may surprise you to learn that the mere act of eating turns up metabolism. When you eat, you stimulate your body to burn energy. Therefore, if you eat smaller, more frequent meals throughout the day, you will burn more energy. Second, your body needs enough amino acids to make muscle and do other essential metabolic tasks. If you don't eat enough protein throughout the day, your level of available amino acids will inevitably drop. If one system within the body needs additional amino acids to function properly, and there aren't enough free amino acids available from your food, it will take what it needs from wherever it can get it, and muscle is one of the richest sources. If you rob your muscles and other storage sites of protein, you will steadily deplete your muscles and bring new muscle production to a grinding halt. On the other hand, if you keep your amino acid levels constant through a steady intake of protein, there will be enough amino acids on hand to do the body's work without wholesale pillaging of your muscles. You may be overwhelmed by the thought of having to eat six meals a day. The fact is, many of you are doing it already, except you don't call it a meal, you call it a snack. I want to change the way you think about food. Every time you put a morsel of food into your mouth, think of it as a meal. It doesn't matter whether it's a handful of peanuts, a doughnut, or a candy bar. It's a meal! The difference is, I'm asking you to put the *right* food into your mouth: protein and fiber. Eating six well-timed meals will help preserve much-needed protein so that you can stay healthy, maintain your muscle, and make new muscle.

Eat More Protein, Burn More Fat

By now you know the Protein Paradox: The more protein you eat, the more fat you burn. That's why I progressively increase your protein consumption over the three cycles of the 6-Pack Prescription Meal Plan and keep you on a moderately high-protein meal plan during your maintenance cycle.

When people begin following the 6-Pack Prescription Meal Plan, they are astonished to find themselves slimming down despite eating more food in general and more protein in particular. I'm not at all surprised. I've worked with thousands of people and have seen the amazing effect of increasing protein consumption on body composition. There is a growing body of scientific evidence proving that protein is a natural fat burner.

Let me tell you about a groundbreaking study I helped to design (conducted at Brigham and Women's Hospital in Boston) of overweight male Cambridge police officers. Like a lot of men their age (28 to 40), these men were beginning to put on weight, lose muscle, and lose strength. Because of their high stress, nonstop lifestyles, they had poor eating habits. For example, many consumed up to 75 percent of their total daily energy intake at dinner. However, they were eating so poorly throughout the day that many of the men were undernourished! Half of these men were already on some kind of weight-loss diet, consuming about 2,200 calories a day, 10 to 20 percent below what their bodies needed. More than 75 percent had a protein intake that was less than the Daily Value—much too little for their physically demanding lives.

In a standard weight-loss program, based on the "You must cut calories to cut fat" formula, these police officers would have been given even *fewer* calories per day to run their bodies. Our study, on the other hand, kept their calorie intake the same while making dramatic changes in their nutrient profile. We fed them more protein.

The police officers were divided into three groups. One group was placed on a diet consisting of the same number of daily calories they had already been consuming (about 80 percent of their daily energy expenditure) and put on a weight-training program. The only change we made in their diet was to increase their protein intake to 25 percent of total daily calories, which typically doubled the amount of protein in their diet. A second group, also on the same number of calories and the same exercise program, was given an additional 70 to 75 grams of protein a day in the form of my specialty protein formula. A third group was given the same basic regimen as the second but with a different protein formula. All three groups lost weight and body fat, despite eating a substantial number of calories. However, the two groups taking the additional protein supplementation lost more weight and, even more importantly, more body fat than the group not taking protein. The group relying on diet alone lost about 2 percent of body fat. The group using the other protein formula lost 4 percent of body fat. The group using my protein formula lost about 8 percent of body fat, or nearly four times that lost by the group on exercise and diet alone! Many of these men were already on a "weight-loss" diet before the study and were getting fatter—

despite eating less than they needed to maintain their body mass. On our regimen with the same number of calories, they lost weight and gained lean mass.

Another recent study, this time of overweight adolescents, proves my point even more dramatically. The kids who were fed 30 percent *more* calories daily, all in the form of protein, lost twice as much body fat as those who were fed a high-carb, low-fat, low-calorie diet. This is a powerful example of nutrient partitioning in practice. When your metabolic traffic cop sees protein coming down the road, he routes it to muscle-building and turns up your fat-burning furnaces. When your metabolic traffic cop sees starchy carbohydrates approaching, he turns the fat-burning furnaces down.

Protein and Fiber: The One–Two Punch Against Fat

While eating more protein will get you in fat-burning mode, eating more fiber will help keep you there. Throughout the three cycles of 6-Pack Prescription, I steadily increase the amount of fiber in your diet until you are consuming 60 grams in the maximum fat-burning phase. Why do we need so much fiber? When fiber is digested, it is fermented in the gut and converted into short-chain fatty acids, which can be burned for fuel. The burning of fatty acids from fiber sends a signal to your fat cells telling them to release fat, which your body uses for fuel. The fiber in food also creates a sensation of feeling full, so you feel more satisfied after eating it. The winning combination of fiber and protein is what kept our cavemen ancestors lean and strong, and it performs the same magic for us.

Unfortunately, fiber has been removed from the modern food supply. Over the past fifty years, modern agriculture has stripped every last bit of fiber out of most of the bread, rice, and cereals sold in grocery stores. Getting rid of fiber is great for manufacturers, because it increases the shelf life of their products, but it's deadly for us. Incredibly, if you want to buy bread with a significant amount of fiber, you have to buy a special loaf to which the fiber has been added back!

The 6-Pack Prescription Meal Plan will show you how to get more fiber back into your diet so that you can take advantage of its fat-burning properties.

Cut Back on Starchy Carbohydrates . . . but You Don't Have to Cut Them Out!

With each cycle of the 6-Pack Prescription Meal Plan, you gradually reduce your consumption of starchy carbohydrates like bread, pasta, and potatoes. Reduce, not eliminate. Even during maximum fat burning (Cycle 3), you will still be able to eat a satisfying amount of starchy carbohydrates. I know that many fad diets today do not allow you to eat starchy carbohydrates at all or have bizarre restrictions; for example, you can't eat them with meat, or you can't eat them with fruit. These approaches are just plain silly. If you like these foods, by all means eat them. You can mix and match them however you like. The protein and fiber in your diet will keep you in fat-burning mode as long as you stay within my carbohydrate guidelines. In the 6-Pack Prescription Meal Plan, I tell you precisely how much of these foods you can eat without getting into trouble. It's a surprisingly large amount.

For those of you who may question whether you can eat any starchy foods and still stay in fat-burning mode, let me tell you about what happens when you simply add protein to the diet of someone eating a large quantity of carbohydrates. You guessed it: They lost fat even with a substantial increase in calories. Researchers added protein to the diets of endurance athletes consuming huge amounts of carbohydrates, the equivalent of ten heaping servings of pasta or a loaf of bread daily. In addition to what they were already eating, half the group was given a daily high-protein beverage, and the other half's diet remained unchanged. At the end of six days, the researchers found that the group getting the extra protein burned fat at twice the rate of the other group and, despite the extra caloric intake, *did not gain an ounce*. I'm not recommending that any of you load up on starch, but you may find it reassuring to know that the moderate amount I allow on the 6-Pack Prescription will not hinder your progress. And having a satisfying diet makes the 6-Pack Prescription an easy meal plan to stay on.

Get the Bad Fats Out of Your Diet

The 6-Pack Prescription allows for a sensible level of fat in your diet. Most of the fat in your diet will be from your protein sources, as protein inevitably contains some fat. There is no reason to count fat grams, but I ask you not to add a lot of extra fat to your food. If you use butter or salad dressing, do so sparingly. I don't want you to eliminate fat from your diet. Fat is an important nutrient: It's essential for many bodily processes. Extremely low-fat diets will dry out your skin and nails, make you tired, and leave you hungry. Too little fat in your diet can slow down fat burning, and that's the last thing we want.

There are many different types of fat in the food that we eat. Some are better for us than others. Dietary fat comes in three varieties: saturated fat, polyunsaturated fat, and monounsaturated fat. The three fats differ in chemical structure, notably in the number of hydrogen molecules. Saturated fats are found primarily in foods of animal origin, like fatty cuts of meat and whole fat dairy products. Plant sources of saturated fat include peanut butter and coconut. Some saturated fats may raise blood cholesterol levels and increase the risk of having a heart attack or stroke. Therefore, I recommend that you limit your intake of saturated fat by sticking to the leanest cuts of meat and low-fat or non-fat dairy products.

Not all saturated fat is created equal. The visible layers of fat outside the actual meat portion, or the muscle, is far worse for you than the fat within the muscle in terms of raising blood cholesterol levels. In fact, some studies suggest that the fat within the muscle of red meat may actually cut cholesterol levels. So, if you eat red meat, be sure to trim off the outer excess fat.

Polyunsaturated fats are found primarily in vegetable oils and margarine made from plant sources. These fats are reasonably healthy in limited quantities, and some of them (safflower oil, canola oil, and sunflower oil) may reduce blood cholesterol levels. They don't, however, have as much flavor as olive oil, a monounsaturated oil that is just as healthy and tastes better. Omega-3 fatty acids found in fatty fish are a special type of polyunsaturated fat that appears to be quite beneficial.

Scores of studies have documented the positive health effects of these fats, which have been shown to lower blood triglyceride levels, reduce the risk of blood clots, and reduce inflammation, and may help prevent certain forms of cancer.

There is one kind of fat I want you to avoid—trans–fatty acids. Some polyunsaturated oils and margarine undergo a process called hydrogenation to make them useful for baking and increase their shelf life. This process creates trans–fatty acids. Trans–fatty acids are living proof of the adage "You are what you eat." Trans–fatty acids may become incorporated within cell membranes, making them rigid, which can interfere with normal cell function. Over time, a diet high in trans–fatty acids can increase your risk of insulin resistance, high cholesterol, and cancer. Trans–fatty acids are found in processed, refined grain products (including cookies, cakes, breads, chips, and other junk foods), and deep-fried foods. Obviously you should steer clear of these fats, but doing that is not as easy as it sounds. As of this writing, the Food and Drug Administration (FDA) does not require manufacturers to list trans–fatty acids on food labels, although the agency is reconsidering that rule. Even though a label may say that a product is cooked in vegetable oil or is low in saturated fat, it may very well contain trans–fatty acids. *Unless a label clearly states that it contains* NO TRANS–FATTY ACIDS, *you have to assume that most processed foods and margarines do.*

Cut the Fructose and the Sugar

In Chapter 3, I asked you to reduce your consumption of high-fructose corn syrup because it is a negative partitioning agent. Please don't get the idea that I think that regular table sugar is fine. Many of us are eating too much sugar in any form. You wouldn't knowingly add 20 teaspoons of sugar to your meals every day, but that's precisely what the average person consumes each day, thanks to hidden sources of sugar. In fact, many people, particularly kids, may unknowingly be eating two to three times that amount—40 to 60 teaspoons of sugar—each and every day! It's been said before but it bears repeating: Avoid foods that contain large amounts of refined sugar.

Sugar produces a tidal wave of glucose that disrupts nutrient partitioning, pushing you into perpetual fat storage. Become vigilant about reading food labels. If you see sugar listed as one of the top three ingredients in a product, consider it a high-sugar food. Look for all forms of sugar, including corn syrup, fruit sugars, and of course high-fructose corn syrup. Sugar will turn up where you least expect it, such as in salad dressings, sauces, canned soups, frozen entrées, and marinades. The occasional use of these products is fine, but if you use several of them every day, you are getting a hefty dose of added sugar.

There are several no-calorie artificial sugar substitutes on the market, two of which I heartily recommend, sucralose and aspartame. The advantage of these sweeteners over sugar is that they do not adversely affect metabolic function. The newest form of sugar is sucralose (sold under the name Splenda), a product made from chemically altered real sugar (sucrose) that cannot be digested by the body. Sucralose tastes like the real thing, can be used like a "tabletop sweetener" by adding it directly to food, or can be used in baking. Sucralose has undergone more than 110 studies in both humans and animals and has proven to be very safe. I am a big fan of sucralose and was one of the first manufacturers to use it in my products. Given the absurdly high amount of sugar consumed in this country, particularly in the form of high-fructose corn syrup, I would like to see sugar replaced by sucralose in such commonly used products as soda.

Aspartame (marketed as NutraSweet and Equal) is another commonly used sugar substitute. Aspartame has been extensively tested and has also been proven to be safe, despite persistent rumors to the contrary. Unlike sucralose, it can't be used in cooking; but it tastes great in iced tea. Use it instead of sugar!

There are other sugar substitutes, but I don't think they are as good as either sucralose or aspartame. Stevia (from the stevia leaf) is a noncaloric sweetener sold primarily in health food stores. It works well as a flavor enhancer in food, but it's not sweet enough for most people to be used as a stand-alone sweetener. Nor has it been approved by the FDA. Other artificial sweeteners include sorbitol (or xylitol), which is nonabsorbable sugar classified as an alcohol. The problem with these sugars is that they can cause stomach upset in many people, so use them with caution.

Food is a powerful tool that can correct the metabolic meltdown that is destroying the health and lives of millions of people of all ages, from the youngest Americans to the oldest. Food can also be a very destructive force. There is no doubt in my mind that eating the wrong food has created the obesity epidemic that is sweeping the country today. And there is no doubt in my mind that eating the right food can stop it. The *Body Rx* approach is a simple one. The 6-Pack Prescription Meal Plan can provide you with the metabolic machinery you need to stay lean, not just for a few weeks or a few months, but for your entire life. Changing how you eat is all it takes to change your body.

I've outlined the basic principles and scientific underpinnings of my program. You now know why it works. Now it's time to make it work for you. In the next chapter, the 6-Pack Prescription Meal Plan, I will give you the specific information you will need to incorporate the meal plan into your life.

In His Own Words

JASON SEHORN

*J*ason Sehorn, star cornerback for the New York Giants, suffered a severe knee injury while returning the opening kickoff in a preseason game. Usually an injury as serious as his would keep a person off the playing field for a year or more after surgery, but not so in Jason's case. Determined to return to the game as quickly as possible, he combined rigorous physical rehabilitation with an eating regimen like that of the 6-Pack Prescription. When Jason reappeared with the Giants for the 1999 season, he was a stronger, leaner, more powerful player who helped lead the team to the 2000 Super Bowl.

I wasn't ready for that injury. I had a clue that it could happen, but you never expect it. When my knee gave way, I said to myself that this was an opportunity to get better, sure, but also to get healthier. I wanted to come back better than when I left. I wanted to work out and stay strong, but I also wanted to do some things differently. So I went to the place with the best support system, and that place was with Dr. Connelly.

When I first met Doc Connelly, I was impressed by how great he looked. He's fifty, but he could pass for thirty. He's in phenomenal

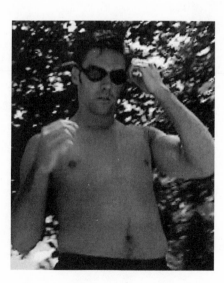
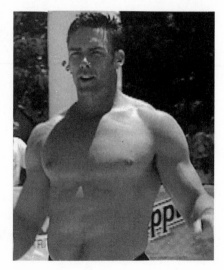

shape. I thought, "Boy, I hope I can look like that when I'm his age." A lot of people can tell you what to do, yet few also practice what they preach. Dr. Connelly's different. Here's a fifty-year-old man who is ripped to shreds, and if he tells me something works, I know it works. I've seen plenty of doctors in my time, but this one talked to me about nutrition and explained what he thought would get the job done, and one glance at him told me that he knew his stuff. From the moment I met him, I considered Dr. Connelly my teacher.

If you want to see changes in your body, you have to eat right and work out. You have to do both. You can't just go to the gym and work out to burn off the calories of junk you just ate—which is what many people do. I learned from Doc Connelly exactly how wrong that is. Every athlete knows how to work out, and every athlete knows how to stay in shape and run and lift. But like everybody else, athletes don't know—really know—about nutrition. Before working with Dr. Connelly, I never understood what good nutrition meant, and I certainly didn't know how important it was. I didn't know what to eat, or when. I'd eat a huge amount and then wait a long time and then eat another large amount. From Dr. Connelly, I learned to eat the right way: eat in increments, eat all day long. He taught me that if you go too long between meals, your body will start storing food because it thinks you're going to starve it. I learned to eat periodically throughout the day. I snack—but not on corn chips or carbs. I grab a nutrition bar or a shake.

I eat out a lot, and that's no problem. Dr. Connelly gave me the tools to eat out without eating wrong. I've been out with him a few times, and I've seen what he does. He'll order something on the menu, but he'll tell the restaurant staff to cook it his way. He'll see chicken with pasta and all this other stuff on the menu, and he'll say, "I want the chicken. Throw the spices on it, but take away the pasta." He doesn't say, "I'll eat around it." He says instead, "Don't even put it on the plate."

So now, at restaurants—and at home—I eat fish and chicken and other lean protein. I stay away from that bread plate that shows up before your order arrives. And I drink water. I don't drink alcohol very often; it's a subtle weight-gain inducer.

There's no doubt in my mind that changing my nutrition has

changed my game. I've worked out my whole life, but until I learned what to put in my body, I wasn't enjoying the maximum effects of those workouts.

The 6-Pack Prescription is not a diet—that's one thing Dr. Connelly has stressed to me. "Don't ever think of this as a diet," he told me. "A diet is temporary. A diet is a short-term goal. What you're doing is a lifestyle change. You're going to do something different from now on." That made sense to me. Because I wasn't going to do this only for a little while. I wanted to change. I wanted to go back to the game better than when I had left it. To get where you want to go, you have to change your habits.

As an athlete, I'm no stranger to discipline and dedication. I know that I won't get what I want without those two things. I have discipline in my training and dedication to my game. You may apply those key ideas to your professional life, to your home, to your goals. Doc Connelly taught me that you need the same discipline and dedication in your nutrition. Without the fundamental fuel for your body, you're not going to reach your goals. A coach once told me that the sad thing about some athletes is that they don't know what they don't know. The same is true of many people and nutrition. If they only stopped to learn what they don't know about nutrition, instead of carrying on as before, they could change their lives.

I give Dr. Connelly a lot of credit for my progress. A transformation took place: I changed my body composition. When I returned to the football field, I was stronger and healthier. I had more power and explosiveness. I'm amazed by how much good came out of the year I spent with Dr. Connelly.

Part II

How to Get the Body You Want

5

The 6-Pack Prescription Meal Plan

Rule No. 1: Food Is No. 1

Food is the number-one tool for transforming your body. To achieve a stronger, sculpted, leaner body, you must give your metabolism the raw materials it needs to start burning fat and building muscle. Expect a lot from your food! Every meal you eat should work with your metabolism, not against it. If you do nothing other than change how and when you eat, you can achieve dramatic results. (If you follow the entire program, you will achieve *spectacular* results.) Eating well is also the key to health. It is the single most important factor in avoiding diabetes, heart disease, high blood pressure, many forms of cancer, and premature aging. In sum, if you want to look and feel terrific, eat as though your life depended on it.

Rule No. 2: Simplicity Rules!

Twenty years' experience of working with thousands of people has taught that when it comes to food, simplicity rules! With rare exceptions, most people eat the same twelve to fifteen foods over and over again, day in and day out. The problem is that we often eat the wrong ones. The 6-Pack Prescription makes it easy for you to switch to the right twelve to fifteen foods. You will choose your favorite foods from my list of high-quality proteins, fruits and vegetables, and breads and starches. You will then design your daily diet around these foods. I have nothing against variety, but through the years I have learned that food plans that are too complicated are unrealistic and doomed to failure. If you're confronted with too many choices or too many things to think about, you'll be tempted to forget about the whole thing. Keep it simple and you will succeed.

Rule No. 3: Eat Often and Eat Enough

Get out of the breakfast, lunch, and dinner rut. *Eat!* Eat six times a day! Eat whenever you are hungry (as long as you eat the right foods). The only way you can cheat on my program is by not eating enough or often enough. Your metabolism works best when it is being fed a steady stream of high-quality fuel. It's essential to eat every two to three hours to keep your metabolism burning fat to build muscle. Skipping meals and cutting calories will not improve your body: It will hinder your fat burning. This is especially true for women, who are natural fat storers. The less often you eat, the more likely your body is to hoard fat. The trick is to load up on foods that stimulate the fat-burning–muscle-building mechanism. You may be thinking, *I don't have time to eat six times a day.* Not so. Eating six meals a day may sound daunting, but actually it's quite simple. In fact, many of you are doing it already but you don't realize it. Every time you pop a snack food or piece of candy into your mouth, you're eating a meal. This all adds up to much more than six meals a day, but your challenge is to make those mini-meals work for you. I will show you how to enjoy six meals of the right stuff!

Rule No. 4: It's About Protein and Fiber

I rely on protein and fiber to keep my body trim and strong, and if you let them, these nutrients can perform the same magic on your body. You need adequate amounts of both to build muscle at the expense of fat. Be vigilant about eating enough high-quality protein and fiber-rich foods. Protein provides the amino acids you need to operate your metabolism and other vital systems. Fiber stimulates fat burning and helps counteract the damaging effects of high-glucose-producing carbohydrates such as grains. This winning combination will keep you sleek and lean.

Rule No. 5: Just Say No to Fructose

Just because food manufacturers put fructose in the food supply doesn't mean that you have to eat it. You don't have to buy, eat, or serve products with a high amount of fructose. Fructose is ubiquitous in food, especially the prepared, processed snacks marketed to children. Read the labels and you will quickly know which products contain fructose and which do not. If you keep your children fructose-free, you will go a long way in helping them to avoid obesity and serious metabolic problems down the road. (This is not a carte blanche to eat sugar. Avoid sucrose as much as possible.)

Rule No. 6: When You Get Control of Your Body, You Get Control of Your Life

It's not just about having a terrific body: It's about achieving your full potential, physically and mentally. Sure, it's wonderful to look in the mirror and think, *I look great*, and that's a given with my program: *You will look great*. But you also gain so much more in the process. You will be empowereed by a newfound confidence, knowing that you radiate health and vitality. You will feel renewed and ready to meet whatever challenges should come your way. You will have the strength and stamina to do things that you once thought were impossible. It doesn't matter whether you're a student, a teacher, a Wall Street trader, a doctor, an Internet billionaire, or a stay-at-home mom. Having a strong body and a sharp mind will better enable you to achieve your goals and fulfill your dreams, not just for the present, but for your future. Remember: If you don't have control over your body, you don't have control over your life. You can keep your body attractive, healthy, and functioning at peak capacity, or you can let it run down, setting yourself up for years of illness and debility. Your health and your destiny are in your hands.

Before You Begin

The 6-Pack Prescription Meal Plan is divided into four six-week cycles and a final six-week maintenance program that you can follow indefinitely. The meal plan is designed to accommodate a wide variety of tastes and eating styles. You can design your menus around the foods that you like. And you won't be a slave to the kitchen. Believe me, I'm not. The meal plan works equally well whether you prepare all your meals at home or eat on the run (as I do).

I wish I could sit down with each one of you and show you how to personalize the program to best suit your needs, as I do with my clients. Obviously that's impossible, but I'm doing the next best thing. Starting on page 92, you will find the 6-Pack Prescription Meal Planner, an easy-to-follow guide that gives you precisely the same tools that I use when I consult one-on-one. The 6-Pack Prescription Meal Planner contains all the information you will need to tailor the meal plan to make it work for you. Your 6-Pack Prescription Meal Planner Part II starting on page 164 includes lists of protein and carbohydrate foods from which to make your daily meal selections. Protein and carbohydrate foods are divided into three different categories: Green foods, Yellow foods, and Red foods.

GREEN MEANS GO! Green foods are the most efficient fat burners. Go for them with abandon. Green carbohydrates include a vast assortment of fruits, vegetables, and two high-fiber cereals. Green carbohydrates are your primary source of fiber. *You can and should eat as many green carbohydrates as you want.*

Green proteins include the leanest cuts of beef, pork, lamb, and poultry, fish, and non- and low-fat dairy products. Not all green proteins are equal. *Super Green proteins are the lowest in fat content.* They include most white-meat poultry, some game meat, fish, and low-fat and nonfat cottage cheese, and exclude beef, lamb, and pork. If you have a high amount of body fat, have a history of heart disease, or want to maintain a "supercut" look, make most of your protein selections from the *Super Green* group. Super Green proteins are designated by an asterisk in the charts on pages 164–165. If you have moderate body fat, are already lean, or are following the program to improve your level of fitness, you can eat freely from any of the Green protein categories.

Remember back in Chapter 1 that I said to stop counting calories? I mean it! The only way you can fail on the 6-Pack Prescription Meal Plan is by not eating your daily requirement of Green and Super Green foods. These are the foods that will keep your metabolism burning fat. I never walk around hungry, and I don't want you to walk around hungry either. When you let yourself get hungry, you get tired and cranky, and end up reaching for the wrong foods, the ones that make you store fat. Moreover, when you get too hungry, it's a signal that your metabolism hasn't been fed often enough to keep it burning at peak efficiency. There's no need to be hungry, as long as you stick to Green foods.

The idea of eating unlimited quantities of food probably goes against everything you've been taught about dieting. I've been teaching the principles of *Body Rx* for the past twenty years, and my major challenge is getting people to abandon the idea that eating until they're full will make them fat. In reality, the opposite is true: *Not eating enough Green foods will make you fat!*

YELLOW MEANS SLOW DOWN! Think of Yellow foods as a yellow light: It's time to slow down. Yellow proteins include cuts of meat, poultry, and dairy products that are higher in saturated fat than Green protein and, therefore, should not be eaten in unlimited quantities.

You may be surprised to see soybean-derived products, such as tofu and tempeh, on the Yellow protein list. In my opinion, soy products do not contain as good an amino acid content as protein derived from animal products. In addition, studies have shown that soy products are also inferior to animal protein when it comes to fat burning. I have another bone to pick with soy: Soy contains high amounts of phytoestrogens, plant chemicals that mimic the effects of the female hormone estrogen in the body. The effects of phytoestrogens are inconclusive. Some studies suggest that they may protect against hormone-sensitive cancers (like breast cancer in women and prostate cancer in men) while others suggest that they may stimulate the growth of tumors. In my opinion, there is ample evidence that these phytoestrogens could actually be harmful to men in terms of promoting fat storage, particularly around the abdomen. Therefore, I advise men to steer clear of soy. Until all the facts are in, I advise people not to consume excess amounts of soy products.

Yellow carbohydrates include all starchy carbohydrates (breads, pasta, cereals, rice, beans) and higher-fat dairy products. For many people following the typical western diet, starchy grains have become the mainstay of their diet. We don't think twice about feasting on a big plate of pasta for dinner, devouring a plate of pancakes for breakfast, grabbing a bagel for a quick snack, or polishing off a basket of bread with dinner. I understand the need to eat pasta, bread, and starch—I like them too—and I know that it's unrealistic to tell people not to eat them. You will anyway, and so will I. I am asking you to cut back to levels that your body can handle. Yellow starches can have a disastrous effect on nutrient partitioning. *The more Yellow carbohydrates you eat, the less fat you will burn.* Eat them in moderation. I will tell you precisely how many portions of Yellow foods are allowed daily in each cycle. Don't worry. It's quite generous, and you won't feel deprived.

Tip for Pasta Lovers

Love pasta? Eat it early in the day. Why? The human body secretes most of its insulin at night, before bedtime, which makes it more likely that starches will be stored as fat. (Remember, pasta is a yellow carbohydrate, so you can't eat it that often.)

RED MEANS STOP! Although there are no forbidden foods on my meal plan, I want you to avoid Red foods as much as possible. Red proteins are high in saturated fat. Red carbohydrates are highly refined, processed foods that are loaded with fructose and sugar but low in fiber. Try to restrict your intake of Red foods to no more than one to two servings a week, and avoid them altogether during Cycle 3, your maximum fat-burning phase.

If Red foods are so bad, why don't I just ban them? I understand that food represents different things to different people. Some people turn to "comfort" foods for emotional solace. Others crave a sugar fix every now and then, and life wouldn't be as much fun without it. Believe me, I understand! I have difficulty walking by a Ben & Jerry's ice cream store without indulging a cone or two, and I don't expect you to give up all the foods that you love either. You should be able to have dessert on the weekend if you really want it. If you're eating at a restaurant known for its cheesecake or "death by chocolate" cake, order it. If you adhere to the principles of the 6-Pack Prescription most of the time, you can indulge yourself on occasion without suffering the consequences.

Keeping Track

The four cycles of the 6-Pack Prescription Meal Plan vary according to the amounts of protein, carbohydrates, and fiber that you will eat daily. As you progress from cycle to cycle, you will eat *more Green foods*—lean protein and good carbohydrates (fruits, vegetables, and high-fiber vegetables) and *fewer Yellow foods* (higher-fat proteins and low-fiber starchy foods.) The amounts of protein and Yellow carbohydrates that you can eat every day depends on your weight. You don't have to get out your calculators: I've worked it all out for you. In your 6-Pack Prescription Meal Planner, you will find Daily Requirement charts that tell you how many grams of protein and Yellow carbohydrates you can eat for each cycle. Some of you don't have to follow the 6-Pack-Prescription Meal Plan down to the last food gram. If you want to buy a food scale and weigh your food, that's fine, but I've never weighed food in my life, I never will, and I don't recommend that you do. You will find it much easier simply to familiarize yourself with the number of protein and carbohydrate grams in the foods that you normally eat. Bear in mind that these are guidelines. Absolute precision is not required. Following my recommendations to a reasonable extent will produce excellent results.

Protein: What's a Portion?

Let me clear up one possible source of confusion. You don't determine the number of protein grams in food simply by weighing it. For example, 8 ounces of steak does not contain 8 ounces of protein. Meat also contains water, fat, and even small amounts of carbohydrate. So how do you figure out the protein content? Actually, it's fairly easy to estimate the number of protein grams in your food. Three ounces of any type of meat, fish, or poultry contains about 20 grams of protein. A 3-ounce portion is roughly the size of a deck of playing cards. Therefore, you can think of 3 ounces—1 deck-size portion—as one 20-gram serving of protein. Remember this simple relationship and you will be able to easily keep track of your protein intake. Of course, the actual serving size that you eat at a given meal may be a lot larger than a deck of cards. The average chicken breast, for example, is roughly the size of two decks of cards. It contains about 40 grams of protein, and thus would count as 2 portions. A cut of steak served at a steakhouse could be the size of four decks of cards, and would count as 4 portions.

> **1 protein portion = 20 grams and is about the size of a deck of cards. Your actual protein serving size per meal = several portions.**

The Daily Requirement chart in your 6-Pack Daily Meal Planner tells you how many protein grams you should eat daily based on your weight for all four cycles. To make it simple, the chart also tells you how many protein *portions* you need to eat for each cycle. For example, if the chart indicates that you need to eat 120 grams of protein daily, you will need to eat six deck-of-card–size portions of lean meat, poultry, or fish. If you divide up your protein requirement over six meals, each serving size per meal would equal 1 portion. If the chart tells you to eat 240 grams of protein daily, you will need to eat twelve deck-of-card–size portions of lean meat, poultry, or fish. If you divide up your protein requirement over six meals, each serving size per meal would be equal to 2 portions. Or, if you eat a particularly large protein meal for lunch (for example, a steak may be equivalent to 4 portions), you may eat a smaller serving of protein for subsequent meals. The point is, once you familiarize yourself with what a protein portion looks like, you can devise the best strategy for fulfilling your daily requirements.

Keeping track of the protein grams in dairy products is also simple. Cottage cheese is the only dairy food that provides a significant amount of protein. One cup of cottage cheese contains 30 grams of protein (1½ portions). If you buy an 8-ounce (1 cup) container of cottage cheese, you don't even have to estimate the portion size. Otherwise, all you have to do is keep in mind that 1 cup of cottage cheese is about the size of your fist. Here are some other rules of thumb: A slice of low-fat cheese weighs about 1 ounce and has about 7 grams of protein. One cup of nonfat yogurt contains about 10 grams of protein (half a portion). If you want exact counts, the number of protein grams are listed on packaged dairy and cheese products.

Counting Carbohydrates

Unfortunately, there is no similarly easy way to measure Yellow carbohydrates, because these foodstuffs come in so many shapes, sizes, and forms! For example, a cup of one brand of cereal could contain 20 grams of carbohydrates, and a cup of another brand could contain twice that amount. Therefore, I have listed the number of carbohydrate grams for particular foods in Part II of your 6-Pack Prescription Meal Planner. You will notice that I do not provide carbohydrate contents for Green carbohydrates. That's because you can eat as many of these as you want. Don't even count them.

Counting Fiber

Most of the fiber in your diet will come from Green carbohydrates or from fiber supplements. Your 6-Pack Prescription Meal Planner Food Guide provides a list of the fiber content of Green carbohydrates. I want you to eat these foods in unlimited quantities because they are the best sources of fiber. Refer to the Food Guide to be sure that you are getting enough fiber every day. As you become more familiar with the fiber content of food, you will soon know that, for example, your favorite salad contains 10 grams of fiber, a medium-size apple contains 4 grams of fiber, your favorite breakfast cereal contains 13 grams of fiber, and so on.

Real-Life Strategies

We don't live in a perfect world where every refrigerator is always fully stocked with the right foods and every meal is eaten on time, around a dining-room table. Today life is more hectic. Most people eat more meals out than they do at home, often under less-than-ideal conditions—in fast-food restaurants, at their desks at work, in hotel rooms, and even in the front seats of their cars. Fortunately, the 6-Pack Prescription Meal Plan is tailor-made for eating on the run, or grabbing a quick meal at home. Here are some techniques that I've developed through years of working with thousands of people to make this program an easy-to-follow way of life.

Protein Strategies

For many people, the major challenge of following my meal plan will be making sure that they meet their daily protein requirement. I know because I do it every day. In Chapter 1, I told you that I practice what I preach. I really do! Most of the time, I follow Cycle 4, the Maintenance Cycle. Since I weigh about 230 pounds, I try to eat about 287 grams of protein daily, or roughly 14 protein portions. (Again, each portion is equivalent in size to a standard deck of cards.) Through the years, I have learned that the easiest way to achieve my nutritional goals is to keep things simple. (Remember: Simplicity rules!) I eat three or four types of protein repeatedly: (1) turkey breast, (2) chicken breast, (3) fish, and (4) steak. I never cook, but I always keep sliced fresh turkey breast and chicken breast in my refrigerator for a quick meal. I buy them at the deli counter at a local supermarket. (I don't buy turkey or chicken roll because they are often filled with additives and loaded with salt.) When I eat out, I usually order grilled swordfish or tuna (my favorite fish) or steak. To make sure I get enough protein, I drink at least two protein shakes daily. (I always order a big salad and lots of grilled vegetables to make sure that I'm also getting enough fiber.)

When eating in a fast-food restaurant, I stick with the program. I scan the menu for the best lean proteins and salads. Nearly all fast-food restaurants offer a version of a grilled chicken sandwich or a plain hamburger, and most have a side salad on the menu. Typically, I'll order two grilled chicken sandwiches and two salads. I then throw away the sandwich buns and put the grilled chicken on the salads. If I'm eating at a sub shop or a deli, I'll order an overstuffed fresh turkey or chicken sandwich with lots of grilled vegetables or lettuce and tomato, and throw away most of the roll.

My protein strategy is easy, uncomplicated, and it works for me.

If you cook, it's even simpler to add protein to your diet. Here are some ways to do that:

- Turn a high-carbohydrate bowl of hot cereal into a high-protein breakfast simply by adding 20 grams of unflavored protein powder to your cooked cereal. (Don't forget to add your extra fiber as well.)

- Add a scoop of protein powder to a serving of sugar-free or plain yogurt or low-fat cottage cheese. Top with fruit or Fiber One cereal for extra fiber. (Fiber One is a Green carbohydrate.)

- Traditional pizza is high in fat and not a great protein source, but with a little bit of help, it can be turned into a great 6-Pack Prescription meal. Instead of regular cheese pizza, order the barbecue (or grilled) chicken pizza and you will greatly enhance the protein content. Use other sources of lean protein (such as lean ham or lean chopped meat) as a topping. At home, you can make your own high-protein pizza. Take a plain ready-made pizza crust, spread your favorite tomato sauce on it, sprinkle on low-fat mozarella cheese, and add a can of white meat chicken or shredded poached or grilled chicken breast. Bake until bubbly hot. Instead of chicken, you can use beanless chili.

• Eat a couple of servings of protein with your salads. Add diced chicken, a can of tuna or salmon, or leftover sliced lean steak.

• Wrap slices of fresh, lean turkey or roast beef in a tortilla and add a salad for a quick meal. Corn tortillas are much higher in fiber.

• Add leftover meats, like lean ham or turkey, to omelettes for added protein and flavor. Eggs are a great source of protein, but they're relatively high in cholesterol (about 300 mg per egg) and contain a fair amount of saturated fat (6 mg per egg), but that doesn't make them bad for you. In fact, several studies have shown that eating eggs even every day does not raise cholesterol levels in healthy people. There is some question as to whether eggs may be harmful for people with existing heart disease. Some people have tried to get around the egg restriction by eating egg-white omelets, or taking one yolk and combining it with several egg whites. This technique not only produces a less tasty omelet but also diminishes the protein value of the eggs. I see no reason to eliminate eggs from your diet, unless you are being treated for high cholesterol and your doctor has told you to do so. For otherwise healthy people, eating several eggs daily is fine.

All About Protein Shakes

Protein shakes are an easy way to make sure that you are meeting your protein requirements for each cycle. Protein shakes can be made from protein powders or purchased as prepackaged protein drinks. Each has its advantages and disadvantages. Protein powders are sold at health food stores, discount pharmacies, and even supermarkets. There are 2 basic types of protein powders:

Total nutrition or complete meal replacement protein. The best meal replacement proteins are derived from a composite of normal milk proteins (casein and whey) and contain at least 30 grams of protein. They also include a complete array of vitamins and minerals, including trace elements. Meal replacement proteins come in different flavors and can be mixed with water or low-fat or nonfat milk (unless you are lactose-intolerant). Many of these products taste pretty good; the only disadvantage is that you don't always have a blender around to mix them. There are several brands to choose from. When you shop for one of these products be sure to look for a label that says TOTAL NUTRITION or COMPLETE MEAL REPLACEMENT PROTEIN on the label.

Pure protein powder. A pure protein powder contains protein and nothing else. A good protein powder provides up to 50 grams of protein per serving. Pure protein powders are useful because they can be made into high-potency protein drinks or used in cooking (e.g., added to oatmeal or casseroles) to enhance the protein content of meals. Pure protein powder is less expensive than the ready-to-drink replacement protein, but remember, it doesn't contain the same full complement of nutrients. I usually recommend that people drink at least one meal replacement drink daily to make sure that they are getting all their nutrients. If you choose to drink an additional protein drink, a pure protein powder is a more economical alternative.

What about people who are lactose-intolerant? Most adults experience some form of lactose intolerance, ranging from the mild to the severe. The lactose content is so minimal in many brands of protein powder that it usually does not cause problems. I should know: I'm lactose-intolerant myself. If you know you are lactose-intolerant, try drinking a small amount of a shake and see if it causes an adverse reaction. In all likelihood you will not have any problems. Don't mix your shakes with milk. Use water. You can also try taking a Lactaid pill before drinking your shake. However, if you are one of those people who cannot tolerate even the tiniest amount of lactose, I recommend that you avoid these products and get your protein from food.

All About Protein Bars

Protein bars (also called food bars, meal replacement bars, and energy bars) can be a convenient and portable way to augment your protein intake on the run. But be very careful: Some protein bars are little more than candy bars in disguise! To make sure that you are getting a high-quality protein bar, read the label. A high-quality protein bar should be at least 30 to 50 percent protein by weight. For example, if the protein bar weighs 100 grams, it should contain at least 30 to 50 grams of protein. Also, beware of added sugar. Shockingly, in the case of many bars, sugar is the first, second, or third ingredient listed on the label. These bars contain a lot more sugar than protein! Also, many protein bars contain high amounts of high-fructose corn syrup. I don't recommend any protein bar in which sugar or high-fructose corn syrup is listed as one of the three top ingredients. For the same reasons mentioned above, I would avoid protein bars in which soy is the primary source of protein. Protein bars do not count in your Yellow carbohydrate totals as long as they have twice the amount of protein as carbohydrates and less than 5 grams of sugar.

Fiber Strategies

Having to double or even triple your fiber intake may be difficult for some of you, but here are some easy ways to get more fiber into your life.

- Make every protein shake a high-fiber shake. Add 1 to 2 teaspoons of sugar-free, unflavored psyllium powder to your shakes before blending. Or add 1 cup frozen or fresh berries (raspberries are highest in fiber) before blending. (Caveat: Ground psyllium seeds from the psyllium plant are a terrific source of fiber but can cause allergic reactions in sensitive people. If you are highly allergic, check with your allergist before using psyllium.)

- Turn ordinary meat loaf, turkey loaf, and casseroles into high-fiber entrees. Replace breadcrumbs with the same amount of Fiber One cereal or rough-cut oatmeal (not the instant kind.)

- If your favorite cereal is not high in fiber, you don't have to give it up. Just add ½ cup of Fiber One or All-Bran to enhance the fiber content.

- Sprinkle high-fiber cereal on sugar-free yogurt or cottage cheese and fresh fruit.

- Eat at least two large, mixed green salads daily. Be sure to include high-fiber vegetables such as peas, tomatoes, peppers, cabbage, and carrots. Romaine lettuce has the highest fiber content of common greens. Make the salad bar one of your regular stops on the way to or home from work.

- Add peppers, onions, and tomatoes to omelettes, sandwiches, and salads.

- Make a quick meal out of freshly cut vegetables and a can of tuna, or fresh turkey or roast beef.

- For a quick mini-meal, grab 2 medium-size apples (8 grams of fiber) and some low-fat cheese sticks. Still hungry? Have a handful of cherries (3 grams of fiber) or a tangerine (3 grams of fiber). See how it all begins to add up?

- Think about fiber content when you select your Yellow carbohydrates. Products vary greatly in fiber content. Some whole-grain bread has 3 to 4 grams of fiber per slice; Italian bread typically has less than 1 gram. You can add 8 grams of fiber to your sandwich simply by selecting the right bread.

- If you don't get enough fiber in your food, use fiber supplements, such as Fibercon or sugar-free Metamucil. Remember, when you use a fiber supplement, you must be vigilant about drinking at least 2 full glasses of water to avoid stomach upset.

- Some people may find that suddenly increasing their fiber intake can cause gastrointestinal discomfort, such as gas and bloating. To prevent problems, introduce fiber slowly, gradually increasing your intake every day. If you've never eaten a high-fiber cereal before, start with ¼ cup and work your way up to ½ cup or a full cup. The same is true for fruits and vegetables. If you rarely eat berries, don't start by eating 3 cups at a time. Start with ½ cup and work your way up to a full cup or more. Before long, your body will get accustomed to more fiber.

An Easy Way to Meet Your Protein and Fiber Targets

For each cycle, do as I do. Try to get at least half your protein and fiber from food, and the rest from supplements.

Fat Strategies

There already is fat in the food you eat. If you follow the 6-Pack Prescription Meal Plan (being careful not to eat too many high-fat proteins) and don't consume too much added fat in your food, you will be eating a healthy level of fat. Here are some things to watch out for:

- Don't add more than 1 to 2 tablespoons of fat (in the form of salad dressings, butter, and other toppings and spreads) to your daily diet.

- Always order salad dressing on the side.

- Cook without added fat: Invest in a good set of non-stick cookware.

- Stick to healthy fats—olive oil and omega-3 fatty acids from fish.

- Avoid trans–fatty acids, which are found in fried and processed foods and some types of margarine.

Eating on the Run

Eating well on the run is a snap, as long as you plan ahead. Stick to the rules—design your meals around protein and fiber—and you will succeed. It's not that hard to do.

- If you eat most of your meals out (as I do), find a nearby deli or restaurant that gives you the best menu options. Keep it simple. Salad bars are great because you can create an easy high-fiber, high-protein lunch simply by adding fresh turkey or chicken or a can of tuna over salad greens. (Avoid pre-made tuna salad and egg salad unless they are made with low-fat mayonnaise.) Grilled lean protein (chicken, fish or a turkey burger) with steamed or grilled vegetables is another great choice, and most menus from coffee shops to fancy restaurants will have something along these lines.

- If you crave a sandwich, by all means eat one, but be sure to keep track of your Yellow carbohydrates. Make sure that the sandwich is positively brimming with the leanest protein (roast beef, turkey, chicken) and that you order mayonnaise on the side. It wouldn't hurt to get a higher-fiber bread, either.

- If you prefer to carry in from Asian restaurants, stick to the basic strategy: Order a dish containing lean protein (chicken, beef, shrimp) served over steamed, fresh vegetables. Be sure it's cooked "clean"—that is, without a heavy, sugary sauce (avoid sweet and sour, for example). In fact, Asian restaurants are a great way of getting your fiber and protein together, as much Asian cuisine is built around this principle. Sushi is fine, too, as long as it's made from more fish than rice.

- If you prefer to brown-bag it, grill an extra portion or two of steak or chicken the night before and bring it to work in a disposable container with leftover salad.

- Keep containers of low-fat cottage cheese, low-fat cheese sticks, and cut-up fresh fruit and vegetables in the office refrigerator. Take some high-fiber cereal to the office. Always keep some ready-to-drink protein shakes or a few protein bars in your desk.

- If your car is your dining room, stock it with the right food. Instead of reaching for junk food, reach for a ready-to-drink protein shake, or a protein bar and a piece of fruit, or a piece of turkey jerky.

What Should I Drink?

Sweetened beverages (like soda, iced tea, and fruit "-ades") are packed with fructose and sugar. These drinks can sabotage your success on this program. I recommend that you drink them only occasionally, if at all.

Water tops my list of preferred beverages. Drink at least 8 glasses of it a day. It helps maintain a favorable hormonal balance in the body that promotes fat burning. If you live in an area where you are concerned about impurities in the water supply, drink bottled water from a reputable company or use a water filter at home.

Real, unsweetened fruit juice is a better alternative to soda, but even the unfiltered stuff is not as good as whole fruit in terms of fiber content. Therefore, I don't recommend that you drink juice every day. Once or twice a week is enough, if you must.

Diet soda is okay if you must drink soda, but soda doesn't count as water. For soda lovers, bubbly water with a twist of lemon or lime is a better choice, and it does count as water.

Alcoholic beverages are high in sugar and should be consumed in limited quantities. I don't drink, but I see nothing wrong with someone having a few drinks a week (not a day!). If you really want to "lean down," however, I would avoid alcohol altogether. Of course, if you have a problem with alcohol, it's best to abstain, as I'm sure you already know.

I don't recommend milk for adults. Milk is a mediocre source of protein, and it contains high amounts of lactose, a sugar that causes gastrointestinal distress in many adults. There are special brands of milk that are lactose-free, and these are better for adults, but I'd suggest getting your dairy from higher-protein forms. Frankly, I prefer that you stick to water. It's fine to use milk in coffee and cereal.

Coffee and tea are also fine if you don't load them up with added sugar. If you must sweeten your coffee or tea, I suggest that you use an artificial sweetener like sucralose or aspartame. Beware of prepackaged coffee and ice tea drinks: They contain high amounts of sugar.

My 6-Pack Prescription
Meal Planner

PART I

My 6-Pack Prescription Meal Planner

Getting Started

You are now ready to customize the 6-Pack Prescription Meal Plan to suit your own body type, food tastes, and lifestyle. The 6-Pack Prescription Meal Planner will guide you through the meal plan, cycle by cycle. In this handy guidebook, you will find the tools you need to ensure your success on the meal plan, including simple charts that will help you customize the program to best suit your needs. Please feel free to make additional copies of these charts as you need them. You may also download additional blank charts from my Web site at www.bodyrxinfo.com.

How to Use the 6-Pack Prescription Meal Planner

Part I of the 6-Pack Prescription Meal Planner is divided into four mini-planners reflecting the different requirements of the four cycles.

Part II of the 6-Pack Prescription Meal Planner contains the lists of Green, Yellow, and Red foods from which you will plan your menus for all four cycles.

Each of the mini-planners begins with a brief description of the goals of the cycle, telling you exactly how much protein and Yellow carbohydrates you should eat, based on your current weight at the beginning of that cycle. (This is the only time you have my permission to step on a scale.) The fiber requirement will be the same for everyone, regardless of weight.

Once you understand these goals, turn to the Daily Requirements chart to determine precisely how many portions of protein and Yellow carbohydrate grams you are allowed for that cycle. No math—I promise! Just look up your numbers, based on your weight.

Turn the page and you will find a handy Daily Tracker. Fill out your personal daily requirements in the box on the upper right-hand side of the page. Use the rest of the chart to keep track of whether you are meeting those goals daily. Fill in your intake of protein portions, fiber grams, and Yellow carbohydrate grams for each of your six meals daily. Add up the total at the end of the day to make sure that you are reaching your goals. Don't go overboard trying to keep track to the last gram, but do try to stay close to your goals. Most of you will need to do this only for about a week at the beginning of each cycle until you become accustomed to your new dietary needs. If you wish to do this for every week, just make copies of the blank chart or download them from my Web site.

Now turn to the chart labeled My Personal Favorites. The best way to succeed at my program is to keep it simple. (Remember: Simplicity rules!) Select six of your favorite proteins, high-fiber Green carbohydrates, and Yellow carbohydrates. Try to plan most of your meals around these foods. You need to keep track of the following three numbers: (1) the fiber content of your favorite Green carbohydrates, (2) the number of fiber grams in your favorite Yellow carbohydrates, and (3) the number of carbohydrate grams in your favorite Yellow carbohydrates. Be sure that you consider the actual serving sizes of your Green and Yellow carbohydrates. For example, a side salad of mixed greens contains around 3 cups of salad greens, but the fiber measurement for salad greens on your Food Chart is for 1 cup. When you eat a salad as a main course, you are actually eating about 4 to 5 cups of salad greens (of course, with added protein). The same is true for many Yellow carbohydrates, like cereal. The Food Chart provides a carbohydrate measure for 1 cup of cereal; you may actually eat 1½ cups of cereal per serving. Take into account your real portion sizes when you record the number of fiber and carbohydrate grams. I've included one chart for each of the four cycles. Not only might your tastes change, but your portion sizes of Yellow and Green carbohydrates will alter as you go through the plan. Take the time to fill out this chart at the beginning of each cycle. It will help you stay on track.

How does all this work? Turn to your Sample Menus, which will show you how easy it is to put simple meals together based on the food charts. After reviewing my sample menus, turn the page and you will see some blank sample menus for you to fill in yourself.

You're ready to get started!

Mini-Planner for Cycle 1: Getting Stronger
(Weeks 1 to 6)

Cycle 1 is designed to ease you into the 6-Pack Prescription Meal Plan. During this cycle, you will probably make a substantial increase in your protein and fiber consumption. However, you won't find yourself missing too many of the yellow carbs you are accustomed to eating. Even though Cycle 1 is going to be an easy transition, you will see substantial changes in your body composition long before six weeks have elapsed. Your body will sport more lean muscle, and the process of shedding fat will be well under way. At the end of this cycle, you should have no doubt that you've made substantial progress, urging you on with every look in the mirror.

During Cycle 1, your goal is to eat 1 gram of protein per pound of body weight daily. For example, if you are a 110-pound woman, you should eat 110 grams of protein; if you are a 180-pound man, you should eat 180 grams of protein. I want you to stick to lean, Green proteins whenever possible, and limit yourself to 3 servings of Yellow proteins a week. If you currently are consuming the typical western diet, which is relatively low in protein and high in starchy yellow carbohydrates, you will find that on my 6-Pack Prescription Meal Plan you will be eating twice the amount of protein that you are accustomed to eating. This should not be difficult. Most people not only like protein foods but actually feel more satisfied when they eat them. For tips on how to get more protein into your diet, see "Protein Strategies" on page 80.

Many readers will not be able to achieve their protein quota on food alone. Protein shakes are an easy and delicious way to get extra protein for all four cycles.

Green carbohydrates are unlimited. For many people, this will mean increasing the amount of healthy fruits and vegetables in their diets, a major side benefit of the 6-Pack Prescription Mean Plan.

During Cycle 1, I want you to restrict your Yellow carbohydrate intake to 2 grams per pound of body weight, up to a maximum of 400 grams daily. This means that a 120-pound woman can eat 240 grams of Yellow carbohydrates, a 180-pound man can eat 360 grams of Yellow carbohydrates, but a 300-pound man tops out at 400 grams of Yellow carbohydrates daily—the maximum allowable. If you are following the standard high-carbohydrate diet, this may be less starch than what you are used to eating, but it is hardly restrictive. Even if what I recommend is less than what you normally eat, given the amount of protein and green carbohydrates you will be eating, you should not feel hungry.

During Cycle 1, regardless of your weight, you should eat 30 grams of fiber. For most of you this will mean doubling the amount of fiber you normally eat.

Now turn to the Daily Requirements chart (pages 97–98) to determine how much protein and Yellow carbohydrates you should eat for this cycle.

MY 6-PACK PRESCRIPTION MEAL PLANNER at a Glance	
(CYCLE 1: GETTING STRONGER)	
Nutrient	**Daily Guidelines**
Protein	**1 gram per pound of body weight measured at beginning of cycle (See Daily Requirements chart for easy reference.)** ✓ Green protein: Make the vast majority of your protein choices from these foods. ✓ Yellow protein: 2 servings per week. ✗ Red protein: Special occasions.
Carbohydrates	**2 grams per pound of body weight measured at beginning of cycle (See Daily Requirements chart for easy reference.)** ✓ Green carbohydrates: Unlimited, does not count toward your total. ✓ Yellow carbohydrates: Stick within your limits. ✗ Red carbohydrates: Special occasions, count toward your limits.
Fiber	**30 grams**

6-PACK PRESCRIPTION DAILY REQUIREMENTS
(Cycle 1: Getting Stronger)

3 ounces of protein = 20 usable grams of protein = 1 portion (roughly the size of a deck of playing cards or an 8–oz protein shake)

Weight	Protein grams	Protein portions	Yellow Carbohydrates grams	Fiber grams
100	100	5	200	30
110	110	6	220	30
120	120	6	240	30
130	130	7	260	30
140	140	7	280	30
150	150	8	300	30
160	160	8	320	30
170	170	9	340	30
180	180	9	360	30
190	190	10	380	30
200	200	10	400	30
210	210	11	400	30
220	220	11	400	30
230	230	12	400	30
240	240	12	400	30
250	250	13	400	30
260	260	13	400	30
270	270	14	400	30
280	280	14	400	30
290	290	15	400	30

6-PACK PRESCRIPTION DAILY REQUIREMENTS
(Cycle 1: Getting Stronger)

3 ounces of protein = 20 usable grams of protein = 1 portion (roughly the size of a deck of playing cards or an 8–oz protein shake)

Weight	Protein grams	Protein portions	Yellow Carbohydrates grams	Fiber grams
300	300	15	400	30
310	310	16	400	30
320	320	16	400	30
330	330	17	400	30
340	340	17	400	30
350	350	18	400	30
360	360	18	400	30
370	370	19	400	30
380	380	19	400	30
390	390	20	400	30
400	400	20	400	30

MY 6-PACK PRESCRIPTION DAILY TRACKER
(Cycle 1: Getting Stronger)

YOUR DAILY REQUIREMENTS

Protein (portions) _____

Fiber (grams) _____

Yellow carbs (grams) _____

Meal	Day 1 Pro	Day 1 Fbr	Day 1 Crb	Day 2 Pro	Day 2 Fbr	Day 2 Crb	Day 3 Pro	Day 3 Fbr	Day 3 Crb	Day 4 Pro	Day 4 Fbr	Day 4 Crb	Day 5 Pro	Day 5 Fbr	Day 5 Crb	Day 6 Pro	Day 6 Fbr	Day 6 Crb	Day 7 Pro	Day 7 Fbr	Day 7 Crb
1																					
2																					
3																					
4																					
5																					
6																					
Totals																					
Goals met?	✓	✓	✓	✓	✓	✓	✓	✓	✓	✓	✓	✓	✓	✓	✓	✓	✓	✓	✓	✓	✓
	✕	✕	✕	✕	✕	✕	✕	✕	✕	✕	✕	✕	✕	✕	✕	✕	✕	✕	✕	✕	✕

MY 6-PACK PRESCRIPTION PERSONAL FAVORITES
(Cycle 1: Getting Stronger)

Protein	Green Carbohydrates	fiber grams	Yellow Carbohydrates	carb grams	fiber grams
1	1		1		
2	2		2		
3	3		3		
4	4		4		
5	5		5		
6	6		6		

Select six of your favorite proteins, high-fiber Green carbohydrates, and Yellow carbohydrates. Try to plan most of your meals around these foods. You need to keep track of the following three numbers: (1) the fiber content of your favorite Green carbohydrates, (2) the number of fiber grams in your favorite Yellow carbohydrates, and (3) the number of carbohydrate grams in your favorite Yellow carbohydrates. Be sure that you consider the actual serving size of your Green and Yellow carbohydrates. Check the food charts beginning on page 164.

SAMPLE MENUS
(Cycle 1: Getting Stronger)
DAY 1

MEAL	MEAL
Low-fat cottage cheese and fresh fruit with Fiber One Coffee or tea	Protein shake
Protein Bar	Lean roast beef sandwich on wheat bread Fresh garden salad with tomatoes Unsweetened iced tea
Roasted turkey and hummus wrap Fresh fruit Sparkling water	Turkey meat loaf Baked potato Steamed assorted fresh vegetables Fresh fruit salad Water

DAY 2

MEAL	MEAL
Scrambled eggs with peppers and scallions Wheat toast Coffee, tea	Barbecued chicken pizza with onions and pepper Fresh fruit
Protein shake	Overstuffed chicken salad sandwich with lettuce and sliced tomato Unsweetened iced tea or diet soda
Low-fat, sugar-free yogurt and fresh fruit	Protein shake

SAMPLE MENUS
(Cycle 1: Getting Stronger)
DAY 3

MEAL	MEAL
Protein bar Coffee or tea	Protein Shake with fiber
Beef jerky Fresh fruit	Baked paprika-crusted chicken breast Mashed potatoes and broccoli Water
Grilled hamburger on a bun with onions, lettuce, and tomato Mixed green salad Unsweetened iced tea or diet soda	Low-fat cottage cheese with fresh fruit and Fiber One

DAY 4

MEAL	MEAL
Protein-enriched apple-spice oatmeal Coffee or tea	Low-fat cheese sticks Fresh fruit
Protein bar	Roasted breast of duck Wild rice pilaf Dinner salad Sparkling water
Chicken cobb salad (chicken breast with mixed greens, hard-boiled egg, and vegetables) Roll Unsweetened iced tea or diet soda	Protein shake with fresh berries

SAMPLE MENUS
(Cycle 1: Getting Stronger)
DAY 5

MEAL	MEAL
Smoked-salmon omelet with dill Whole wheat toast Coffee or tea	Protein shake with raspberries
Protein bar Red pepper spears	Low-fat grilled cheese sandwich with tomatoes and onions Mixed green salad Unsweetened iced tea or diet soda

Chef salad (white turkey slices, low-fat
    cheese over mixed greens and vegetables,
    dressing on the side)
Sparkling water
	Grilled swordfish with spicy fruit salsa
	Steamed asparagus
	Fruit salad
	Water

DAY 6

MEAL	MEAL

English muffin, egg, and low-fat cheese
    sandwich
Fresh fruit
Coffee or tea
	Grilled chicken breast over a Caesar salad
	    (dressing on the side)
	Dinner roll
	Diet soda

Low-fat cottage cheese with fresh fruit	Protein bar with fruit
Protein shake	Beef stir-fry with mixed steamed vegetables over white sticky rice Water

SAMPLE MENUS
(Cycle 1: Getting Stronger)
DAY 7

MEAL	MEAL
Protein-enriched oatmeal with nutmeg and sliced apple Coffee or tea	Protein bar
Low-fat cheese sticks Fresh fruits	Pork tenderloin with baked apples Dinner salad Dinner roll Glass of white wine or sparkling water
Waldorf salad (grilled chicken over greens, green and red apples, with raspberry vinaigrette) Unsweetened iced tea or diet soda	Protein shake with fiber

BLANK MENUS
(Cycle 1: Getting Stronger)

DAY 1	
MEAL	**FOOD**
1	
2	
3	
4	
5	
6	

BLANK MENUS
(Cycle 1: Getting Stronger)

DAY 2

MEAL	FOOD
1	
2	
3	
4	
5	
6	

BLANK MENUS
(Cycle 1: Getting Stronger)

DAY 3	
MEAL	**FOOD**
1	
2	
3	
4	
5	
6	

BLANK MENUS
(Cycle 1: Getting Stronger)

DAY 4

MEAL	FOOD
1	
2	
3	
4	
5	
6	

BLANK MENUS (Cycle 1: Getting Stronger)	
DAY 5	
MEAL	FOOD
1	
2	
3	
4	
5	
6	

BLANK MENUS
(Cycle 1: Getting Stronger)

DAY 6	
MEAL	**FOOD**
1	
2	
3	
4	
5	
6	

BLANK MENUS
(Cycle 1: Getting Stronger)

MEAL	FOOD
DAY 7	
1	
2	
3	
4	
5	
6	

Mini-Planner for Cycle 2: Getting Sculpted
(Weeks 7 to 12)

During Cycle 2, you will be working on developing better muscle definition, and my meal plan will help you achieve those goals. You will increase your protein intake from 1 gram to 1.25 grams per pound of body weight per day. Essentially what this means is that you will be eating an additional protein portion daily. (See charts on pages 113–115.) Make most of your selections from the lean, Green protein list, and reduce the amount of fattier, Yellow proteins to 1 serving a week.

Green carbohydrates remain unlimited. You will reduce your Yellow carbohydrate intake from 2 grams to 1 gram per pound of body weight, with a maximum of 400 grams per day. You are not going to feel deprived. For example, a 100-pound woman can still eat 100 grams of Yellow carbohydrate foods each day. This is the equivalent of 2 slices of bread plus a cup of pasta.

During Cycle 2, I want you to increase your fiber intake to 45 grams daily.

Now turn to your Daily Requirements chart to determine how much protein and Yellow carbohydrates you should eat for this cycle.

MY 6-PACK PRESCRIPTION MEAL PLANNER at a Glance	
(CYCLE 2: GETTING SCULPTED)	
Nutrient	**Daily Guidelines**
Protein	**1.25 grams per pound of body weight measured at beginning of cycle (See Daily Requirements chart for easy reference.)** ✓ Green protein: Make the vast majority of your protein choices from these foods. ✓ Yellow protein: 1 serving per week. ✗ Red protein: Special occasions.
Carbohydrates	**1 gram per pound of body weight measured at beginning of cycle (See Daily Requirements chart for easy reference.)** ✓ Green carbohydrates: Unlimited, does not count toward your total. ✓ Yellow carbohydrates: Stick within your limits. ✗ Red carbohydrates: Special occasions, count toward your limits.
Fiber	**45 grams**

6-PACK PRESCRIPTION DAILY REQUIREMENTS
(Cycle 2: Getting Sculpted)

3 ounces of protein = 20 usable grams of protein = 1 portion (roughly the size of a deck of playing cards or an 8–oz protein shake)

Weight	Protein grams	Protein portions	Yellow Carbohydrates grams	Fiber grams
100	125	6	100	45
110	137	7	110	45
120	150	8	120	45
130	162	8	130	45
140	175	9	140	45
150	187	9	150	45
160	200	10	160	45
170	212	11	170	45
180	225	11	180	45
190	237	12	190	45
200	250	13	200	45
210	262	13	200	45
220	275	14	200	45
230	287	14	200	45
240	300	15	200	45
250	312	16	200	45
260	325	16	200	45
270	337	17	200	45
280	350	18	200	45
290	362	18	200	45

6-PACK PRESCRIPTION DAILY REQUIREMENTS
(Cycle 2: Getting Sculpted)

3 ounces of protein = 20 usable grams of protein = 1 portion (roughly the size of a deck of playing cards or an 8–oz protein shake)

Weight	Protein grams	portions	Yellow Carbohydrates grams	Fiber grams
300	375	19	200	45
310	387	19	200	45
320	400	20	200	45
330	412	21	200	45
340	425	21	200	45
350	437	22	200	45
360	450	23	200	45
370	462	23	200	45
380	475	24	200	45
390	487	24	200	45
400	500	25	200	45

MY 6-PACK PRESCRIPTION DAILY TRACKER
(Cycle 2: Getting Sculpted)

YOUR DAILY REQUIREMENTS

Protein (portions) _____

Fiber (grams) _____

Yellow carbs (grams) _____

Meal	Day 1 Pro	Day 1 Fbr	Day 1 Crb	Day 2 Pro	Day 2 Fbr	Day 2 Crb	Day 3 Pro	Day 3 Fbr	Day 3 Crb	Day 4 Pro	Day 4 Fbr	Day 4 Crb	Day 5 Pro	Day 5 Fbr	Day 5 Crb	Day 6 Pro	Day 6 Fbr	Day 6 Crb	Day 7 Pro	Day 7 Fbr	Day 7 Crb
1																					
2																					
3																					
4																					
5																					
6																					
Totals																					
Goals met?	✓	✓	✓	✓	✓	✓	✓	✓	✓	✓	✓	✓	✓	✓	✓	✓	✓	✓	✓	✓	✓
	✕	✕	✕	✕	✕	✕	✕	✕	✕	✕	✕	✕	✕	✕	✕	✕	✕	✕	✕	✕	✕

MY 6-PACK PRESCRIPTION PERSONAL FAVORITES
(Cycle 2: Getting Sculpted)

Protein	Green Carbohydrates	fiber grams	Yellow Carbohydrates	carb grams	fiber grams
1	1		1		
2	2		2		
3	3		3		
4	4		4		
5	5		5		
6	6		6		

Select six of your favorite proteins, high-fiber Green carbohydrates, and Yellow carbohydrates. Try to plan most of your meals around these foods. You need to keep track of the following three numbers: (1) the fiber content of your favorite Green carbohydrates, (2) the number of fiber grams in your favorite Yellow carbohydrates, and (3) the number of carbohydrate grams in your favorite Yellow carbohydrates. Be sure that you consider the actual serving size of your Green and Yellow carbohydrates. Check the food charts beginning on page 164.

SAMPLE MENUS
(Cycle 2: Getting Sculpted)
DAY 1

MEAL	MEAL
Scrambled eggs with low-fat turkey sausage Coffee or tea	Protein drink with fresh berries
Protein bar with fresh fruit	Low-fat cheese sticks Fresh fruit
Sliced roasted turkey sandwich with avocado and tomatoes Garden salad Unsweetened iced tea or diet soda	Grilled marinated beef kabobs with tomatoes, pepper, and onion Garlic couscous Water

DAY 2

MEAL	MEAL
High-fiber sugar-free cereal with fresh fruit and skim milk Coffee or tea	Balsamic grilled chicken breast sandwich on seven-grain bread with onions and tomatoes Garden salad Unsweetened iced tea or diet soda
Low-fat cottage cheese with fresh berries	Protein bar with fresh fruit
Protein drink with fresh fruit	Grilled red snapper with steamed asparagus Dinner salad Water

SAMPLE MENUS
(Cycle 2: Getting Sculpted)
DAY 3

MEAL	MEAL
Southwestern omelet (avocado, low-fat cheddar cheese, tomato, and salsa) Fresh fruit Coffee or tea	Grilled hamburger patty with melted low-fat cheese and sliced tomato Garden salad Unsweetened iced tea or diet soda
Protein drink	Protein bar
Teriyaki beef jerky Fresh fruit	Spicy chicken stir-fry with steamed vegetables and white sticky rice Water

DAY 4

MEAL	MEAL
Protein-enriched oatmeal with fresh blueberries Coffee or tea	Blackened chicken Caesar salad Unsweetened iced tea or diet soda
Nonfat, sugar-free yogurt with Fiber One Fresh fruit	Protein drink
Protein bar Fresh fruit	Filet mignon with baked potato Steamed artichoke Dinner salad Water

SAMPLE MENUS
(Cycle 2: Getting Sculpted)
DAY 5

MEAL	MEAL
Omelet with smoked ham, green peppers, and onions Whole wheat toast Coffee or tea	Low-fat cottage cheese with Fiber One and melon
Protein drink with fresh fruit	Protein bar with fresh fruit
Greek salad with herbed chicken sausage Dinner salad Unsweetened iced tea or diet soda	Meat loaf with grilled portobello mushrooms Garlic mashed potatoes Garden salad Sparkling water

DAY 6

MEAL	MEAL
Low-fat cottage cheese with Fiber One and fresh fruit Coffee or tea	Hawaiian pizza with smoked ham and pineapple Mixed green salad Diet soda
Low-fat cheddar cheese with sliced apples Wheat crackers	Baked lobster tail with garlic oil Steamed broccoli with lemon Dinner salad Water
Protein drink with fresh fruit	Protein bar

SAMPLE MENUS	
(Cycle 2: Getting Sculpted)	
DAY 7	
MEAL	**MEAL**
Protein shake with fresh fruit Coffee or tea	Tex-Mex chicken salad (spicy grilled chicken over mixed greens, salsa, and low-fat cheddar cheese) Garden salad Unsweetened iced tea or diet soda
Low-fat cheese sticks Fresh fruit	Protein drink with fresh berries
Low-fat cottage cheese with Fiber One	Grilled sirloin steak with sauteed onions and garlic Baked yam Dinner salad with pea pods 1 glass of red wine or water

BLANK MENUS
(Cycle 2: Getting Sculpted)

DAY 1	
MEAL	**FOOD**
1	
2	
3	
4	
5	
6	

BLANK MENUS
(Cycle 2: Getting Sculpted)

DAY 2	
MEAL	**FOOD**
1	
2	
3	
4	
5	
6	

BLANK MENUS (Cycle 2: Getting Sculpted)	
DAY 3	
MEAL	**FOOD**
1	
2	
3	
4	
5	
6	

BLANK MENUS
(Cycle 2: Getting Sculpted)

DAY 4	
MEAL	**FOOD**
1	
2	
3	
4	
5	
6	

BLANK MENUS (Cycle 2: Getting Sculpted)

DAY 5	
MEAL	FOOD
1	
2	
3	
4	
5	
6	

MEAL	FOOD
BLANK MENUS (Cycle 2: Getting Sculpted)	
DAY 6	
1	
2	
3	
4	
5	
6	

BLANK MENUS
(Cycle 2: Getting Sculpted)

DAY 7	
MEAL	**FOOD**
1	
2	
3	
4	
5	
6	

Mini-Planner for Cycle 3: Burning Fat
(Weeks 13 to 18)

During Cycle 3, you will burn fat at a blistering pace. You will boost your protein intake to 1.5 grams of protein per pound of body weight daily. (See the charts on pages 130–132.) During this cycle, I want you to eat the leanest proteins and avoid Yellow and Red proteins entirely.

During Cycle 3, you will reduce your consumption of Yellow carbohydrates to 0.5 grams per pound of body weight. This is a lot less starch than you may be used to eating, but it's not punishing. You can still eat 2 to 3 servings of starchy foods. It won't seem like much of a step down after you've gradually reduced your intake in cycles 1 and 2. In fact, by this point, many of the people I work with have dropped their Yellow carb intake to this level naturally.

During Cycle 3, you will increase your daily fiber intake to 60 grams. That may be a lot for some of you, and frankly, I know that some of you won't make it every day. But remember, that fiber burns fat, and that's why I'm asking you to eat so much of it during this critical last phase.

Now turn to your Daily Requirements chart to determine how much protein and Yellow carbohydrates you should eat for this cycle.

MY 6-PACK PRESCRIPTION MEAL PLANNER
at a Glance

(CYCLE 3: BURNING FAT)	
Nutrient	**Daily Guidelines**
Protein	**1.5 grams per pound of body weight measured at beginning of cycle (See Daily Requirements chart for easy reference.)** ✓ Green protein: Make the vast majority of your protein choices from these foods. ✗ Yellow protein: none. ✗ Red protein: none.
Carbohydrates	**1 gram per pound of body weight measured at beginning of cycle (See Daily Requirements chart for easy reference.)** ✓ Green carbohydrates: Unlimited, does not count toward your total. ✓ Yellow carbohydrates: Stick within your limits. ✗ Red carbohydrates: none.
Fiber	**60 grams**

6-PACK PRESCRIPTION DAILY REQUIREMENTS
(Cycle 3: Burning Fat)

3 ounces of protein = 20 usable grams of protein = 1 portion (roughly the size of a deck of playing cards or an 8–oz protein shake)

Weight	Protein grams	Protein portions	Yellow Carbohydrates grams	Fiber grams
100	150	8	50	60
110	165	8	55	60
120	180	9	60	60
130	195	10	65	60
140	210	11	70	60
150	225	11	75	60
160	240	12	80	60
170	255	13	85	60
180	270	14	90	60
190	285	14	95	60
200	300	15	100	60
210	315	16	100	60
220	330	17	100	60
230	345	17	100	60
240	360	18	100	60
250	375	19	100	60
260	390	20	100	60
270	405	20	100	60
280	420	21	100	60
290	435	22	100	60

6-PACK PRESCRIPTION DAILY REQUIREMENTS
(Cycle 3: Burning Fat)

3 ounces of protein = 20 usable grams of protein = 1 portion (roughly the size of a deck of playing cards or an 8–oz protein shake)

Weight	Protein grams	portions	Yellow Carbohydrates grams	Fiber grams
300	450	23	100	60
310	465	23	100	60
320	480	24	100	60
330	495	25	100	60
340	510	26	100	60
350	525	26	100	60
360	540	27	100	60
370	555	28	100	60
380	570	29	100	60
390	585	30	100	60
400	600	31	100	60

MY 6-PACK PRESCRIPTION DAILY TRACKER
(Cycle 3: Burning Fat)

YOUR DAILY REQUIREMENTS

Protein (portions) _____

Fiber (grams) _____

Yellow carbs (grams) _____

Meal	Day 1			Day 2			Day 3			Day 4			Day 5			Day 6			Day 7		
	Pro	Fbr	Crb	Pro	Fbr	Crb	Pro	Fbr	Crb	Pro	Fbr	Crb	Pro	Fbr	Crb	Pro	Fbr	Crb	Pro	Fbr	Crb
1																					
2																					
3																					
4																					
5																					
6																					
Totals																					
Goals met?	✓	✓	✓	✓	✓	✓	✓	✓	✓	✓	✓	✓	✓	✓	✓	✓	✓	✓	✓	✓	✓
	✕	✕	✕	✕	✕	✕	✕	✕	✕	✕	✕	✕	✕	✕	✕	✕	✕	✕	✕	✕	✕

MY 6-PACK PRESCRIPTION PERSONAL FAVORITES
(Cycle 3: Burning Fat)

Protein	Green Carbohydrates		fiber grams	Yellow Carbohydrates		carb grams	fiber grams
1	1			1			
2	2			2			
3	3			3			
4	4			4			
5	5			5			
6	6			6			

Select six of your favorite proteins, high-fiber Green carbohydrates, and Yellow carbohydrates. Try to plan most of your meals around these foods. You need to keep track of the following three numbers: (1) the fiber content of your favorite Green carbohydrates, (2) the number of fiber grams in your favorite Yellow carbohydrates, and (3) the number of fiber and carbohydrate grams in your favorite Yellow carbohydrates. Be sure that you consider the actual serving size of your Green and Yellow carbohydrates. Check the food charts beginning on page 164.

SAMPLE MENUS
(Cycle 3: Burning Fat)
DAY 1

MEAL	MEAL
High-fiber, sugar-free cereal with fresh fruit and skim milk Coffee or tea	Protein drink with fiber
Protein bar Fresh fruit	Low-fat cottage cheese with Fiber One and blueberries
Hamburger patty with sautéed onions on a toasted bun Mixed green salad Unsweetened iced tea or diet soda	Roasted turkey breast with sliced tomatoes Garden salad with pea pods Water

DAY 2

MEAL	MEAL
Protein-enriched oatmeal with cinnamon and sliced apples Coffee or tea	Soy-ginger chicken salad with mandarin orange Unsweetened iced tea or diet soda
Nonfat sugar-free yogurt with added fiber Fresh fruit	Salade Niçoise (white-meat tuna over greens, hard-boiled egg, and string beans, with a vinaigrette) Water
Protein drink Melon medley	Protein bar with fresh fruit

SAMPLE MENUS
(Cycle 3: Burning Fat)
DAY 3

MEAL	MEAL
Whole grain toast Shrimp omelet with tarragon Coffee or tea	Protein drink with fiber
Protein bar Fresh fruit	Sliced lean roast beef with gravy Steamed broccoli Dinner salad Water

Grilled chicken breast with
    artichoke hearts
Unsweetened iced tea or diet soda
	Low-fat unsweetened yogurt with
	    Fiber One
	Water

DAY 4

MEAL	MEAL
Protein drink with fiber Coffee or tea	Protein drink with frozen berries
Turkey jerky Fresh fruit Unsweetened iced tea or diet soda	Seared scallops with spaghetti squash Dinner salad Water
Chicken Caesar salad with onions, red and green peppers Roll Unsweetened iced tea or diet soda	Protein bar Water

SAMPLE MENUS
(Cycle 3: Burning Fat)
DAY 5

MEAL	MEAL
Poached eggs on sourdough toast Fresh fruit Coffee or tea	Protein drink with frozen berries
Protein drink with added fiber	Grilled filet mignon with sautéed onions and mushrooms Dinner salad Water
Teriyaki turkey burger with sliced pineapple Mixed green salad Unsweetened iced tea or diet soda	Protein bar with fresh fruit

DAY 6

MEAL	MEAL
Low-fat cottage cheese with fruit and Fiber One Coffee or tea	Protein bar with fresh fruit
Protein drink with added fiber	Homemade beef chili Dinner salad Water
Grilled salmon with mustard sauce Tomato and basil salad Unsweetened iced tea or diet soda	Protein drink with fresh berries

SAMPLE MENUS
(Cycle 3: Burning Fat)
DAY 7

MEAL	MEAL
Cheddar cheese omelet with onions and red peppers Whole wheat toast Coffee or tea	Marinated tuna steak with ginger Chinese cabbage Water
Protein bar Fresh fruit	Blackened chicken salad Fresh fruit
Grilled chicken and portobello mushrooms in wine sauce Grilled vegetables Unsweetened iced tea or diet soda	Protein drink with fiber

BLANK MENUS
(Cycle 3: Burning Fat)

DAY 1	
MEAL	FOOD
1	
2	
3	
4	
5	
6	

BLANK MENUS	
(Cycle 3: Burning Fat)	
DAY 2	
MEAL	FOOD
1	
2	
3	
4	
5	
6	

BLANK MENUS
(Cycle 3: Burning Fat)

DAY 3	
MEAL	**FOOD**
1	
2	
3	
4	
5	
6	

BLANK MENUS
(Cycle 3: Burning Fat)

DAY 4

MEAL	FOOD
1	
2	
3	
4	
5	
6	

BLANK MENUS	
(Cycle 3: Burning Fat)	

DAY 5	
MEAL	**FOOD**
1	
2	
3	
4	
5	
6	

BLANK MENUS
(Cycle 3: Burning Fat)

DAY 6	
MEAL	**FOOD**
1	
2	
3	
4	
5	
6	

MEAL	FOOD
BLANK MENUS (Cycle 3: Burning Fat)	
DAY 7	
1	
2	
3	
4	
5	
6	

Mini-Planner for Cycle 4: Maintenance and Endurance
(Week 19 to 24)

Congratulations! You've made it through the first three cycles of the meal plan, and you should feel proud of yourself for your accomplishment. By now, you're reaping the rewards of eating well. By the time you have completed Cycle 3, your body will be stronger, shapelier, and leaner, and you will want to keep it that way. During Cycle 4, the maintenance phase, you will eat 1.25 grams of protein per pound of body weight. You can eat up to 4 servings of yellow proteins per week and 1.5 grams of yellow carbohydrates per pound of body weight per day. It's still a good idea to reserve Red foods for special occasions, but eating them once or twice a week is fine.

The maintenance cycle is especially easy to follow because each week you get to "take one day off" and eat whatever you want. In fact, these "days off" are an important part of the program. The radical departure from your normal eating style turns up your fat-burning machinery. It gives your metabolism a good workout. It's also psychic nutrition: Knowing that you can give into your food cravings one day a week can keep you in tow the other six.

You know the drill. . . . Turn to Your Daily Requirements chart to determine how much protein and Yellow carbohydrates you should eat for this cycle.

MY 6-PACK PRESCRIPTION MEAL PLANNER
at a Glance

	(CYCLE 4: MAINTENANCE)
Nutrient	Daily Guidelines
Protein	**1.25 grams per pound of body weight measured at beginning of cycle (See Daily Requirements chart for easy reference.)** ✓ Green protein: Make the vast majority of your protein choices from these foods. ✓ Yellow protein: 4 servings per week. ✕ Red protein: Special occasions.
Carbohydrates	**1.5 grams per pound of body weight measured at beginning of cycle (See Daily Requirements chart for easy reference.)** ✓ Green carbohydrates: Unlimited, do not count toward your total. ✓ Yellow carbohydrates: Stick within your limits. ✕ Red carbohydrates: Special occasions, count toward your limits.
Fiber	**50 grams**

6-PACK PRESCRIPTION DAILY REQUIREMENTS
(Cycle 4: Maintenance)

3 ounces of protein = 20 usable grams of protein = 1 portion (roughly the size of a deck of playing cards or an 8–oz protein shake)

Weight	Protein grams	Protein portions	Yellow Carbohydrates grams	Fiber grams
100	125	6	150	50
110	137	7	165	50
120	150	8	180	50
130	162	8	195	50
140	175	9	210	50
150	187	9	225	50
160	200	10	240	50
170	212	11	255	50
180	225	11	270	50
190	237	12	285	50
200	250	13	300	50
210	262	13	300	50
220	275	14	300	50
230	287	14	300	50
240	300	15	300	50
250	312	16	300	50
260	325	16	300	50
270	337	17	300	50
280	350	18	300	50
290	362	18	300	50

6-PACK PRESCRIPTION DAILY REQUIREMENTS
(Cycle 4: Maintenance)

3 ounces of protein = 20 usable grams of protein = 1 portion (roughly the size of a deck of playing cards or an 8–oz protein shake)

Weight	Protein grams	Protein portions	Yellow Carbohydrates grams	Fiber grams
300	375	19	300	50
310	387	19	300	50
320	400	20	300	50
330	412	21	300	50
340	425	21	300	50
350	437	22	300	50
360	450	23	300	50
370	462	23	300	50
380	475	24	300	50
390	487	24	300	50
400	500	25	300	50

MY 6-PACK PRESCRIPTION DAILY TRACKER
(Cycle 4: Maintenance)

YOUR DAILY REQUIREMENTS

Protein (portions) _____

Fiber (grams) _____

Yellow carbs (grams) _____

Meal	Day 1			Day 2			Day 3			Day 4			Day 5			Day 6			Day 7		
	Pro	Fbr	Crb	Pro	Fbr	Crb	Pro	Fbr	Crb	Pro	Fbr	Crb	Pro	Fbr	Crb	Pro	Fbr	Crb	Pro	Fbr	Crb
1																					
2																					
3																					
4																					
5																					
6																					
Totals																					
Goals met?	✓	✓	✓	✓	✓	✓	✓	✓	✓	✓	✓	✓	✓	✓	✓	✓	✓	✓	✓	✓	✓
	✕	✕	✕	✕	✕	✕	✕	✕	✕	✕	✕	✕	✕	✕	✕	✕	✕	✕	✕	✕	✕

MY 6-PACK PRESCRIPTION PERSONAL FAVORITES
(Cycle 4: Maintenance)

Protein	Green Carbohydrates	fiber grams	Yellow Carbohydrates	carb grams	fiber grams
1	1		1		
2	2		2		
3	3		3		
4	4		4		
5	5		5		
6	6		6		

Select six of your favorite proteins, high-fiber Green carbohydrates, and Yellow carbohydrates. Try to plan most of your meals around these foods. You need to keep track of the following three numbers: (1) the fiber content of your favorite Green carbohydrates, (2) the number of fiber grams in your favorite Yellow carbohydrates, and (3) the number of fiber and carbohydrate grams in your favorite Yellow carbohydrates. Be sure that you consider the actual serving sizes of your Green and Yellow carbohydrates. Check the food charts beginning on page 164.

SAMPLE MENUS
(Maintenance Meal Plan)
DAY 1

MEAL	MEAL
Tuna salad and hard-boiled egg over crudité Fresh orange Coffee or tea	Nonfat yogurt Fresh fruit
Protein shake and berries	Rotisserie chicken Steamed vegetables Baked potato Fresh fruit salad Water
High-fiber cold cereal with milk Mineral water	Protein shake

DAY 2

MEAL	MEAL
Low-fat cottage cheese, fresh fruit, and Fiber One cereal Coffee or tea	Protein shake and berries
Hard-boiled egg Fresh fruit salad	Chicken or shrimp with Chinese vegetables Rice Nonfat chocolate pudding Mineral water
Turkey burger on a whole grain bun Green salad Iced tea	Low-fat cheese sticks Fresh fruit

SAMPLE MENUS
(Maintenance Meal Plan)
DAY 3

MEAL	MEAL
Protein-enriched oatmeal Fresh fruit Coffee or tea	Protein bar Fresh fruit
Protein shake and berries	Baked fillet of sole stuffed with crabmeat Unsweetened iced tea
Turkey sandwich on rye with lettuce and tomato Coleslaw Watermelon Diet soda	Low-fat cheese sticks Apple

DAY 4

MEAL	MEAL
Vegetable omelet Whole grain toast Coffee or tea	Protein shake and berries
Unsweetened yogurt with fresh fruit, and Fiber One	Dill poached salmon Grilled vegetables Steamed orzo Mineral water
Grilled chicken pizza Salad Iced tea	Protein bar Fresh fruit

SAMPLE MENUS
(Maintenance Meal Plan)
DAY 5

MEAL	MEAL
Low-fat cheese slices and lean ham Wasa crackers Cantaloupe and fresh blueberries Coffee or tea	Low-fat cottage cheese and Fiber One
Protein shake and berries	Flank steak teriyaki Steamed broccoli Whole wheat couscous
Chicken fajitas (grilled chicken and vegetables in a fajita wrapper) Fresh fruit Iced tea	Protein bar Apple

DAY 6

MEAL	MEAL
Ham and cheese omelet Whole grain toast Fresh fruit cup Coffee or tea	Protein bar and fruit
Protein shake and berries	Grilled halibut Stir-fried vegetables Dinner roll Glass of white wine
Steak salad (leftover flank steak on greens)	High-fiber cereal with milk and fresh fruit

SAMPLE MENUS
(Maintenance Meal Plan)
DAY 7 IS A FREE DAY

MEAL	MEAL

FREE DAY

BLANK MENUS
(Cycle 4: Maintenance)

DAY 1

MEAL	FOOD
1	
2	
3	
4	
5	
6	

BLANK MENUS
(Cycle 4: Maintenance)

DAY 2

MEAL	FOOD
1	
2	
3	
4	
5	
6	

BLANK MENUS
(Cycle 4: Maintenance)

DAY 3	
MEAL	**FOOD**
1	
2	
3	
4	
5	
6	

BLANK MENUS
(Cycle 4: Maintenance)

DAY 4	
MEAL	**FOOD**
1	
2	
3	
4	
5	
6	

BLANK MENUS (Cycle 4: Maintenance)	
DAY 5	
MEAL	**FOOD**
1	
2	
3	
4	
5	
6	

BLANK MENUS (Cycle 4: Maintenance)	
DAY 6	
MEAL	**FOOD**
1	
2	
3	
4	
5	
6	

	BLANK MENUS (Cycle 4: Maintenance)
	DAY 7
MEAL	**FOOD**
1	
2	
3	
4	
5	
6	

FREE DAY

My 6-Pack Prescription
Meal Planner

PART II

GREEN PROTEIN

3 ounces of protein = 20 usable grams of protein = 1 portion (roughly the size of a deck of playing cards or an 8–oz protein shake)

BEEF (USDA select or choice grades of meat, trimmed of fat)

Beef tenderloin	Filet mignon	Sirloin steak
Cubed steak	Flank steak	Veal roast
Ground round, lean	Round steak	Veal chop, lean
Ground sirloin, lean	Roast beef (top round or rump)	

LAMB

Chop	Roast	Leg

PORK

Canadian bacon	Loin chop	Sausage (less than 1 gram of fat per ounce)
Lean ham (boiled, canned, or baked)	Pork tenderloin	

POULTRY

Chicken, white meat, no skin*	Ground turkey*	Deli meats made from chicken or turkey (95% fat-free)
Cornish hen, no skin*	Chicken or turkey hot dogs or sausage (less than 3 grams of fat per ounce)	
Turkey, white meat*		
Ground chicken*		

GAME

Buffalo*	Goose, without skin	Rabbit
Duck (well drained of fat, no skin)	Ostrich	Venison*
	Pheasant	

*Super Green foods.

GREEN PROTEIN

3 ounces of protein = 20 usable grams of protein = 1 portion (roughly the size of a deck of playing cards or an 8–oz protein shake)

FISH *(grilled, broiled, or baked; fresh or frozen)*

Bass*	Mackerel	Scallops*
Bluefish	Orange roughy*	Shrimp*
Catfish	Oysters	Swordfish steak
Cod*	Perch*	Trout
Crab	Pike*	Tuna (canned in water
Flounder*	Pollock*	or fresh)*
Haddock*	Scallops*	Turbot*
Herring (uncreamed)	Snapper (red or yellow)*	Whitefish*
Halibut*	Salmon (canned in water	
Imitation shellfish	or fresh)	
Lobster	Sardines (canned)	

DAIRY

Eggs	Cheese with 3 grams of	Grated Parmesan (2 table-
Nonfat or low-fat	fat or less per slice	spoons per portion)
cottage cheese*		

*Super Green foods.

YELLOW PROTEIN

3 ounces of protein = 20 usable grams of protein = 1 portion (roughly the size of a deck of playing cards or an 8–oz protein shake)

BEEF

All grades of prime beef	New York strip	T-bone steak
Corned beef	Porterhouse steak	Veal cutlet (cubed or unbreaded)
Ground beef (chuck)	Short ribs	

LAMB

Rib roast	Ground

PORK

Top loin	Pork chop	Sausage (5 grams of fat or less per ounce)
Boston butt	Pork cutlet	

POULTRY

Chicken, dark meat	Turkey, dark meat

FISH

Fried fish of any kind

DAIRY

Cheese (5 grams of fat or less per ounce)	Feta cheese	Ricotta cheese
	Mozzarella cheese	

SOY

Soy milk	Tempeh	Tofu

RED PROTEIN

3 ounces of protein = 20 usable grams of protein = 1 portion (roughly the size of a deck of playing cards or an 8–oz protein shake)

BEEF

Sandwich meats (bologna, pimiento loaf, salami with 8 grams or more of fat per ounce)	Brisket Full-fat beef hot dogs (6–8 grams of fat per ounce)	Prime rib roast Rib steak

PORK

Bacon Bratwurst Full-fat pork hot dogs (6–8 grams of fat per ounce)	Ground pork Knockwurst Pork sausage (Italian, Polish)	Spareribs

POULTRY

Fried chicken	Chicken nuggets	Chicken Parmesan

DAIRY

All regular full-fat cheeses (American, cheddar, Monterey Jack, Swiss)

NUTS

All nuts	Nut butters

Fiber Content of Foods	
Green Carbohydrates	**Fiber grams**
Grains	
All-Bran cereal *(1 cup)*	31
Fiber One cereal *(1 cup)*	28.5
Fruits	
Apple *(1 medium)*	4
Applesauce, unsweetened *(1 cup)*	3
Apricots, fresh	2
Avocado *(1 medium)*	10
Banana *(1 medium)*	3
Blackberries *(1 cup)*	8
Blueberries *(1 cup)*	4
Boysenberries *(1 cup)*	5
Cantaloupe *(½ melon)*	2
Cherries *(10 fresh)*	3
Fig *(1 raw)*	2
Mango *(½ small)*	2
Nectarine *(1 medium)*	2
Papaya *(1 cup)*	2.5
Peach *(1 medium)*	2
Pear *(1 medium)*	4
Persimmon *(1 medium)*	6
Pineapple *(1 cup)*	2
Plum *(1 small)*	1
Pomegranate *(1 medium)*	1
Raspberries *(1 cup)*	8
Strawberries *(1 cup)*	4
Tamarind *(1 raw)*	5
Tangerine *(1 medium)*	2
Watermelon *(1 slice, or ¹⁄₁₆ melon)*	1.5
Vegetables *(1 cup raw or ½ cup cooked)*	
Artichoke hearts	6
Arugula	0.5

Fiber Content of Foods	
Green Carbohydrates	**Fiber grams**
Vegetables *(1 cup raw or ½ cup cooked)* *(continued)*	
Asparagus *(6 spears cooked)*	1.5
Bamboo shoots	3
Bean sprouts	1
Beets	4
Bell peppers	2
Bok choy	1
Broccoli	3
Brussels sprouts	3
Cabbage	2
Carrots	4
Cauliflower	2.5
Celery	2
Cucumber	1
Endive	1.5
Eggplant	2
Fennel bulb	3
Jerusalem artichokes	2
Jicama	6
Kale	1.5
Kohlrabi	5
Leeks	2
Mushrooms	1
Mustard greens	2
Okra	3
Onion	3
Parsnips	7
Peas in the pod	2
Radishes	2
Salad greens	1
Sauerkraut	3.5
Scallions	3
Snow peas	2

Fiber Content of Foods	
Green Carbohydrates	**Fiber grams**
Vegetables *(1 cup raw or ½ cup cooked)* *(continued)*	
Spinach	1
String beans	4
Sugar snap peas	2
Summer squash	2
Tomato	2
Tomato, canned	2
Tomato sauce	3.5
Turnips	2.5
Water chestnuts	3
Watercress	0.5
Zucchini	1.5

Fiber and Carbohydrate Contents of Foods

Yellow Carbohydrates	Fiber grams	Carb grams
Starchy Vegetables		
Acorn squash. *(1 cup cooked)*	9	29
Beans, *lentil, pinto, black* *(1 cup cooked)*	16	40
Butternut squash *(1 cup cooked)*	6	24
Corn on the cob *(1 ear)*	4	30
Hummus (*mashed chickpeas*) *(1 cup)*	15	36
Idaho potatoes *(1 medium)*	2.5	34
Potato, mashed *(1 cup)*	4	35
Pumpkin *(1 cup cooked)*	3	12
Sweet potato *(1 medium)*	3.5	28
Yukon gold potato *(1 medium)*	2.5	34
Yams *(1 medium)*	5.5	38
Breads and Crackers		
Animal crackers *(8)*	0.22	15
Bagel *(3½ inches across) plain, poppy, sesame, etc.*	2	38
Bread, white *(1 slice)*	0.5	13
Bread, whole wheat *(1 slice)*	2	13
Bread, rye *(1 slice)*	2	15.5
Bread, Italian *(4 inches long)*	1	15
Bread crumbs *(1 cup)*	1	22
Bread sticks *(4 by ½ inches)*	0.15	3.5
Bun, hamburger or hot dog *(1 roll)*	1	22
English muffin *(1 muffin)*	1.5	26
Graham crackers *(1 square)*	0.19	5
Matzo *(1 piece)*	1.5	22
Melba toast *(4 slices)*	1.25	15
Oyster crackers *(24 crackers)*	1	17
Pita *(6 inches across)*	1.5	33.5
Pizza crust *(½ 6-inch pie)*	3	32
Rice cakes *(4 inches across, 2 cakes)*	0	20

Yellow Carbohydrates	Fiber grams	Carb grams
Breads and Crackers *(continued)*		
Roll, plain small	1	14
Saltines *(2 crackers)*	0.18	4
Tortilla, corn *(6 inches across)*	1.5	12
Tortilla, wheat *(7–8 inches across)*	1.5	27
Wasa crisp bread *(3 crackers)*	2	11
Wasa flat bread *(3 crackers)*	2	11
Whole wheat crackers *(2 crackers)*	0.25	4
Cereals *(1 cup cooked or ready to eat)*		
Granola *(low fat)*	6	80
Grape-Nuts	10	94
Grits	0.5	31
Kashi	2	13
Muesli	6.5	56
Oatmeal *(100 grams)*	2.5	16
Puffed cereals	0.25	13
Shredded wheat	5.5	40
Special K	1	22.5
Wheat germ	14.5	56
Wheatena	6.5	29
Wheaties	2.1	24
Grains *(1 cup cooked)*		
Amaranth	30	129
Barley	6	44
Bulgur	8	34
Couscous	2	36.5
Kamut	1	23
Kasha *(buckwheat)*	4.5	33.5
Millet	2.5	39
Pasta *(regular)*	2.5	39
Pasta *(artichoke)*	1	41
Pasta *(spinach)*	3	37

Yellow Carbohydrates	Fiber grams	Carb grams
Grains *(continued)*		
Rice *(white)*	0.5	44.5
Rice *(brown)*	3.5	45
Quinoa	10	117
Wild rice	3	35
Snack Foods		
Popcorn *(3 cups)*	4.25	22
Potato chips **(light)** *(15–20 chips)*	0	17
Pretzels *(¾ ounce)*	1	17

Our food supply is so packed with refined, processed and highly sweetened food products that it is virtually impossible to list all Red carbohydrates. Given the variety of products and brands, the list would be longer than this book! Therefore, I have narrowed down the list to general categories of the most commonly consumed Red carbohydrates.

Because you are not going to eat Red carbohydrates more than once a week, you don't have to worry about keeping track of them as closely as you do for Yellow carbohydrates. Nevertheless, I want you to be aware of their carbohydrate content. Because there are so many different products, I can't list each and every product with its carbohydrate count. For your convenience, I have compiled a chart that you can use as a quick reference for most Red carbohydrates. It's not exact, but it's within the ballpark. For the precise count, be sure to check the package for the exact carbohydrate content.

RED CARBOHYDRATES
QUICK REFERENCE CHART

1 small (1 ounce) bag of chips	15 grams
2 sandwich cookies or 4 single small cookies or 1 small brownie	20 grams
1 slice of plain cake or toaster pastry	35 grams
1 slice of cake with icing	40 grams
1 slice of pie with top and bottom crust	40 grams
1 slice of pie without top crust	30 grams
1 cup of fruit ice	50–60 grams
½ cup of ice cream	20 grams
½ cup of frozen yogurt	25 grams
1 can of soda	40 grams

RED CARBOHYDRATES

Snack Foods

Chips (potato, corn, cheese-flavored, etc.)

Granola bars

Breakfast bars

Toaster pastry

Presweetened Cereals

All varieties

Desserts

All cake (chocolate, coffee cake, cheesecake, etc.)

All pies

Cookies (all varieties)

Cupcakes

Ice cream (full-fat and nonfat)

Frozen yogurt

All candy (chocolate, fruit-flavored, caramel, jelly beans, etc.)

Fruit snacks

Fruit rolls

Sorbet

Fruit ice

Presweetened packaged puddings (artificially sweetened Jell-O and pudding are okay)

Marshmallows

Condiments

Maple syrup

Catsup with fructose

Honey (pure fructose: use sparingly)

Molasses

Beverages

All non-diet soda

Presweetened tea and fruit drinks

Hot chocolate

Presweetened coffee drinks

Mixed alcoholic beverages

Beer

Wine

Malted milk

Milk shakes

6

Body R~x~: Exercise

The 6-Pack Prescription Workout provides a specific, targeted weight-training program that can create a lean, strong body. Why weight training? *Weight training is the only exercise that can produce significant changes in your body composition.* If you follow my program, you will make more muscle and lean mass, and you will lose body fat. I believe that you will also enjoy yourself in the process.

Why not aerobics? In all honesty, I detest doing aerobics. To me, running aimlessly on a treadmill or stomping on a stair stepper is mind numbing. Running in place or climbing a stairway to nowhere? Those are the epitomes of futility! But that's not why I don't recommend aerobics for others. The benefits of aerobics pale in comparison to those of weight training. In terms of health benefits, *weight training does everything that aerobics can do, and much, much more.*

For those of you who may be unfamiliar with exercise terms, aerobic activities (like running and jogging) involve large amounts of muscle mass that are exercising continuously at an intensity level that uses primarily oxygen as the gasoline, the fuel source. In contrast, anaerobic exercising (like weight training, sprinting) are short-term activities that can be so intense, they exceed the body's capability to utilize oxygen, so the body must also burn other forms of fuel, such as glycogen, which is stored carbohydrate in muscle.

Aerobic exercise is sometimes referred to as "cardio" because your heart rate increases during your workout. When done regularly, aerobics train your heart and lungs to pump blood more efficiently to your maximal point, which varies from person to person. This is often referred to as your aerobic capacity, or in scientific terms, your maximal oxygen uptake. The more aerobic capacity you have, the greater your endurance and the longer you can exercise. That's great, but it has no bearing on your heart health. The common misconception persists that aerobic exercise gives your heart a better workout than weight training. Contrary to popular opinion, the cardiovascular benefit of aerobics is not due to its direct action on your heart. Rather, it is due to its effect on blood pressure. Aerobic exercise relaxes the outer arteries delivering blood to your muscle cells. There are trillions of tiny arteries feeding your muscles, and when they are dilated (relaxed), your blood pressure drops, resulting in a greater flow of oxygen-carrying blood to be delivered to your muscles. This allows your heart to become more efficient in delivering oxygen to your body to fuel exercise. Despite all the hype about aerobics being essential for you heart, the truth is, *you can get exactly the same benefit from weight training.* Weight training relaxes those same tiny arteries, lowering your blood pressure just as surely. Moreover, there are many other benefits that you get from weight training that you don't get from aerobics.

Aerobics does nothing to help you build muscle mass and strength (in fact, high-intensity aerobics may even reduce muscle mass and strength), and at the end of the day, that's what counts. If you are trying to recomposition your body, muscle is the *only* thing that counts. It can turn you into a champion fat burner and give you a strong and sculpted body. The weight room is the only place you can build muscle, and with the help of your new diet, you'll be building it at a remarkable pace. (See "Making Muscle, Burning Fat" below.)

You've undoubtedly heard the expression "use it or lose it." This is a particularly apt description of what happens to muscle. From age 30 on, if we do nothing to stop it, we will lose an average of 2 to 4 pounds of muscle each decade. At the same time you're losing muscle, you may also be losing bone, as in the case of osteoporosis. The loss of muscle begins a downward spiral, leading to the eventual frailty and wasting syndrome seen in the elderly. This dismal scenario need not happen! Weight training is the only exercise that can save and repair your muscles and build bone so that you stay straight and stay strong for your entire life. Having a great aerobic capacity will not help you retain muscle mass or keep you out of a nursing home later in life. It doesn't even guarantee that you won't have a heart attack! If you have limited time to spend at the gym, don't squander it on aerobics. Spend it wisely in the weight room. I know that there are people who really love doing aerobics, and if you're one of them, go ahead and do them, but only as an adjunct to weight training, not as a substitute.

I have worked with many people, particularly women, who have been doing aerobics for years with little or no result. The more time they spend on the treadmill, the less improvement they see. When asked why they keep doing something that seems so ineffective, their usual response is "I'm afraid if I stop doing it, I'll get fat." Of course they will: Their faulty nutrient-partitioning systems are keeping them locked in fat-storage mode, and the constant aerobics aren't doing much to help. They're running in place instead of moving forward. Once I get them off the treadmill and into the weight-training room, they begin to understand what the right exercise program can do for them.

Not everyone has had a successful experience with weight training. Many people have said to me, "I've worked with weights before and it didn't do anything for me." When I watch them at the gym, I can see why: They're doing it all wrong! The key to effective weight training is to work with the right intensity. Many people mistakenly believe that the right way to lift weights is to do endless repetitions with very low weights. Instead of increasing weight as their workout gets easier, they keep increasing their repetitions. This is not only extraordinarily time-consuming but extraordinarily ineffective. Weight training is called *progressive* resistance for a reason: You're supposed to make progress! I'm not talking about lifting so much weight that you get hurt, but I *am* talking about lifting enough weight to challenge your muscles with each workout. My program shows you how to continually increase your weights so that you get excellent results, safely and quickly.

Let me dispel one of the major myths about weight training. First, many women worry that lifting heavy weights will make them big and muscular like men. This is simply not true. Women do not have the same hormones as men and cannot get as big as men no matter how hard they work out. Lifting heavy weights will produce bigger muscles, but muscle is more compact than fat. The end result is a more defined body, not a bigger one. That bears repeating: Muscle is so much more compact than fat that increasing your muscle size at the expense of your fat will inevitably result in a smaller body. In fact, the woman in the exercise photos you'll see in the next chapter is a wonderful example of this in action. While you'll read her story later, let me give you a preview. Before she became conscious of her body composition, Deb had gone from a size 12 to a size 8 as a result of conventional dieting. While she was thinner than she had been in a long time, it took a grueling low-calorie regimen to keep her there. Once she started on the 6-Pack Prescription Workout, Deb dropped to a size 2 (without dieting). She is by all measures smaller, trimmer, and healthier, despite having considerably more muscle than before. I guarantee that if you measure the size of your waist or thigh six weeks after beginning a weight-training program, it will be getting smaller, not bigger. At the end of six weeks, you will be wearing a smaller size, just like Deb.

Making Muscle, Burning Fat

The positive effects of a well-designed weight-training program are far-reaching and long lasting. The process of making and maintaining muscle has a nearly magical effect on the body. It is a true rejuvenator in every sense of the word. The most obvious effect is cosmetic. Within a few weeks, you will look slimmer and leaner both in your clothes and out of them. Lean muscle is the body's main vehicle for fat burning, and by increasing your amount of muscle, you are not only eliminating existing fat but also drastically decreasing the chances of getting fat in the future.

The term *making muscle* is actually a misnomer because you are born with all the muscle cells that you are ever going to have. Unlike other cells in your body, which can replicate themselves, muscle cells lose the ability to reproduce while you are still in the womb. But muscle cells have a special talent: They are designed to repair themselves when they are injured, resulting in a bigger, stronger cell. If you sustain an injury to a muscle, your muscle cells will come back better than before. It's how your body was designed to adapt itself to changing circumstances. This principle underlies weight training. When you lift a heavy weight, you cause microscopic injury to your muscle cells. The injury triggers a chain of beneficial events that make your muscles bigger and stronger.

If you look at a muscle cell under a high-powered electron microscope, you will see large, dark chromatic dots, or satellite cells outside the cell membrane, which encases the cell. These satellite cells are actually dormant reserves of DNA, genetic material that can make cells grow. When a muscle cell is injured, the cell membrane releases special growth factors called IGF-1 and IGF-2. When a satellite cell comes in contact with IGF-1, it begins to replicate its DNA, producing a new, immature muscle cell similar to the cells found in fetuses. Then IGF-2 sends a signal telling the cells to stop replicating, and the new immature cells begin to develop into mature muscle fibers. The satellite cell extends a cytoplasmic bridge to an adjacent, mature fiber and the two fuse along the entire cell membrane. What you now have is a bigger, thicker, stronger muscle cell. By the way, this process can be activated throughout your entire life span. I have a slide of a satellite cell merging with a mature muscle cell taken from a 99-year-old man! The body has a remarkable capacity to repair and enlarge muscle cells at any age: There are trillions and trillions of satellite cells, most of which will remain dormant unless we call them to action.

Don't worry, you don't have to hurt yourself to trigger the repair response. The act of lifting and lowering a challenging weight is all it takes to stimulate this wonderful process of muscle renewal. But that's not all it does. At the same time, you are also consuming a huge amount of energy. In fact, from an energy standpoint, the process of making muscle and maintaining muscle is very expensive. First, constructing new muscle tissue consumes an enormous amount of energy. Second, since muscle is more metabolically active than fat tissue, it requires a great deal of energy to sustain it. Thus, *the more muscle you have, the more fat you will burn, not only during times of activity, but during times of rest.*

Making Champion Fat-Burning Cells

Weight training offers another extraordinary benefit: It can make your muscle cells better fat burners. Although everyone is born with roughly the same amount of muscle cells, the type and composition of muscle cells vary from person to person. Some people may be genetically blessed with muscle cells that are better fat burners.

There are two types of muscle fibers, fast-twitch fibers and slow-twitch fibers. You are stuck with the ones you were born with. Slow-twitch muscle fibers are the fibers used for endurance activities, like running a marathon. These fibers are great at fat burning. Fast-twitch muscle fibers are the kind of muscle cells used for weight lifting and holding your body up against gravity. These fibers are sluggish fat burners. You can have an amount of muscle identical to the next person's, but if you've been blessed with a high percentage of slow-twitch fibers, you'll be a much better fat burner. If you've been dealt more fast-twitch fibers, you won't burn as much fat.

But there is something you can do about it. Weight training can improve the fat-burning efficiency of fast-twitch muscle cells. Even if you were born with muscle cells that are poor fat burners, you can get the same—or even better—metabolic spin as a person born with slow-twitch cells by weight training, and weight training alone. Aerobics doesn't do this.

Do It Right!

In order to achieve the benefits of weight training, you need to do it with enough intensity that your muscles are getting a true workout. The injury-repair mechanism that makes bigger and better muscles will not be activated unless you give your muscles a sufficient challenge. Simply increasing your repetitions without increasing your weight is a waste of your time. If you want results, do it right! The instructions, charts, and photos in the next chapter will walk you through the 6-Pack Exercise Plan. If you follow the weight-training program, you will be continually challenging your muscles, building a tighter body, and turning yourself into a champion fat burner.

The Synergy Between Nutrition and Weight Training

Both making muscle and maintaining muscle require a greater expenditure of energy, which will increase fat burning. If you provide the body with the right fuel mix—fiber for fatty acids and protein to make lean mass—the entire cost of making and maintaining muscle will be paid for by your fat stores. With proper nutrition, you don't have to lose one ounce of your lean mass to make bigger and better muscles.

In Her Own Words

DOTTIE A. LESSARD-O'CONNOR

Dottie A. Lessard-O'Connor, who underwent a double lung transplant in 1994, is a certified fitness trainer and a multiple medal winner at the 1998, 1999, and 2000 U.S. Transplant Games. By any standard, she is an exceptionally strong and fit athlete. For someone with cystic fibrosis, she is positively remarkable. Once given little hope by her doctors of surviving, much less having a normal existence, Dottie is living an extraordinary life today. She is married, training for a triathlon, writing a book, and operating Dottie's Dream, a nonprofit organization that provides exercise equipment to children three to eighteen years old with cystic fibrosis who are awaiting or who have already received a lung transplant. Dottie lives with her husband, John O'Connor, in Bradford, Massachusetts. From her story, you can see that exercise and proper nutrition constitute powerful medicine.

I was diagnosed with cystic fibrosis when I was still a baby, but I stayed fairly healthy until my teens. I had some shortness of breath when I tried to run, but all in all, I was able to lead a normal life. Even though I couldn't do what most other kids could do, I always considered myself a

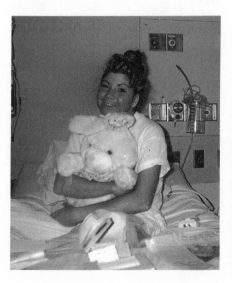
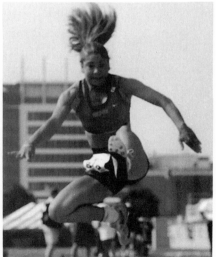

tomboy. Things changed when I was fifteen. I noticed I couldn't ride my bike as fast as before, and I started having coughing fits that left me short of breath. Soon I had my first "cleanout"—I had to go to the hospital to have the mucus cleaned out of my lungs. From then on, I spent most of my school vacations in the hospital having a cleanout. Despite these treatments, I could tell things were getting worse. I started to measure the distance betweeen one classroom and another. My close friends knew I had CF, but I never wanted to be pitied or treated differently from others. I tried to hide it as much as I could. I'd take a lot of trips to the bathroom—that's where I had my coughing fits.

After graduation, everybody was going off to college, and I wanted to do so as well. I went to a two-year college for an associate's degree in fashion merchandising and design. That way I could still live at home. It was hard. I needed physical therapy every day to clear my chest. I couldn't do much exercise, but in 1986, when a boyfriend of mine said girls couldn't do it, I began lifting weights. His comment made me angry, so my dad gave me some hand weights, and I started with them. From the minute I picked up a weight I loved it; I wouldn't be as short of breath as I would with other exercise, and I felt I was doing something good for myself.

I graduated from college, but I wasn't healthy enough to get a job. I spent a lot of time at home, trying not to let myself get any sicker. Nevertheless, by 1992, I was going into the hospital every few months for a cleanout. I would be in for two weeks, then home for a couple of months, then in again. I felt I was just existing and not living. I couldn't go out with friends. If I went to the mall with my mother, I'd sit on a bench with old ladies while she shopped. It was depressing for a girl my age, and particularly difficult for one who always wanted to be healthy and athletic.

My future looked bleak. I was put on a list for a double lung transplant in May 1992. I'm five-foot-four and weighed only 101 pounds, and the doctors warned me that if I lost any more weight, I'd need a feeding tube. I then started reading everything I could on fitness and nutrition. I tried weight-gain drinks, but none of them helped. They all tasted bad, and they felt heavy in my stomach. When I had coughing fits, the drinks would come right back up. One day I opened a fitness magazine and came across an article about Dr. Connelly and the protein drink he had invented. What he said in the article about the importance of nutrition and the right protein made so much sense to me. A lot of doctors don't pay attention to nutrition, they focus on the illness. But if your nutrition is off, so is everything else. I started drinking Dr. Connelly's protein formula, and within three months I went from a frail 101 pounds to a healthy 115. And I didn't gain fat, I gained muscle. In 1994, before my transplant surgery, the doctors who did the medical workup thought they were looking at the wrong CT scan. They said I had an incredible amount of muscle mass for someone with my condition.

When I had the transplant surgery, the doctors knew I was sick, but they did not realize what bad shape my lungs were in; my muscles had adapted. I did not need oxygen before my transplant, while many people in my situation do. I think my lungs adapted to what little I could give them because my body was in good condition. When the doctors opened me up, my lungs were a lot worse than my overall condition had led them to believe. I died twice on the table. I had to be on a heart-lung machine, and the surgery took twelve hours. I remember my surgeon coming in after the operation. "Thank you for saving my life," I told him. And he said, "Well, I didn't save your life, you did—by keeping yourself in shape." I'll never forget that. I really did fight hard, working out and paying attention to nutrition, but I don't think I would be here today without Dr. Connelly.

In 1998, a few years after my transplant, I participated in the U.S. Transplant Games. I had no idea what to expect. I'm proud to say that I came in fourth in the 100 meters and won a silver medal in the long jump. I couldn't run so much as a block before, and here I was competing! The next year, I won a gold medal in the long jump, a silver in the 100 meters, and a bronze in the softball throw. In 2000, I won a gold medal for both the 100 and the 200 meters.

I don't take anything for granted. I continue to care for myself and drink my protein shakes. I look forward to a long, full life. My husband and I want to buy a house and start a family. All of these things would have seemed impossible ten years ago, when I wasn't even sure whether I would survive surgery. Today, I can see myself living to be eighty, watching my grandchildren play on the front lawn. I am passionate about fitness and nutrition—I would not be here without them.

7

The 6-Pack Prescription Workout

> - *Exercise each muscle group only once a week.*
>
> - *Do only five exercises at a time.*
>
> - *Exercise only four days a week.*
>
> - *Do your workouts on your own schedule.*
>
> - *No aerobics required!*
>
> - *Get great results in six weeks.*

The 6-Pack Prescription Workout is a simple and easy way to organize your workout regimen. There are twenty basic weight training exercises, divided into four separate workout sessions, each to be performed once a week. In other words, I'm asking you to exercise only four days a week. Each session consists of five exercises and should take

186

about one hour from start to finish. As with the food plan, the 6-Pack Prescription Workout is divided into four six-week cycles. Each cycle has the same goals as it did in the food plan: getting stronger, getting sculpted, burning fat, and maintenance and endurance. Each of the four cycles uses the same exercises, but the amount of weight, number of repetitions, and length of resting periods between sets vary from cycle to cycle. A repetition is defined as one complete lift and return of the weight. A set is a group of repetitions performed without a rest.

The 6-Pack System enables you to design your workout regimen to best suit your schedule. Since you exercise each muscle group only once a week, you'll only have to spend four days working out each week. Moreover, unlike most other plans, you don't need a day or two to recover between each session because the muscles you used the previous day won't be used again for a week. The next day you are on to another muscle group. If you like, you can exercise four days in a row, every other day, or twice on the weekends and twice during the week. The program is flexible enough to adapt to even the busiest or most erratic schedules.

You'll see a full description of the exercises later in this chapter. I've included pictures and easy-to-follow instructions to help you become comfortable with these movements, even if you've never done them before. You'll also find a flexible exercise schedule. I don't care what time of day you exercise or what days you choose to work out. However, I do ask that you do the exercises in the order I've laid them out. On your first exercising day of the week, you'll work your chest and biceps, doing exercises 1 to 5 in order; Day 2 is back and triceps; Day 3 is legs, hamstrings, and calf muscles; and Day 4 is shoulders and abdominal muscles. By the end of the week, you should have covered every muscle group.

There is a specific strategy to the order of the exercises in each session. The first two to three exercises in each day's program are designed to engage as much muscle mass as possible. By doing this, you exercise the major muscle groups before they get too fatigued from stabilizing other movements to get a good workout. The last two to three exercises focus on smaller, accessory muscle groups, which should not be too tired from the previous exercises for an effective workout. I've designed this plan so that you do not exercise complementary major muscle groups on the same day: That can diminish the effectiveness of your workout. For example, you won't work your chest and shoulders on the same day, since when you work your chest, you are also using your shoulders. My aim is to give you the most time-efficient workout possible, and you get that from using fresh, rested muscles.

My program is designed to achieve the fastest results in the shortest period of time. It is extraordinarily efficient and works equally well for both beginners and advanced weight trainers. If you've been spending a lot of time working out with no discernible benefits, I urge you to give my method a try.

Nearly all of the exercises in the 6-Pack Prescription Workout are to be performed on exercise machines that can be found at most major gyms and health clubs. In instances when a machine is hard to come by, however, I recommend using free weights. For some exercises, I've illustrated both machine and free-weight versions. Pick whichever one suits you best. For the beginner, I recommend exercise machines over free weights. Exercise machines are safer for beginning weight lifters. Working with free weights requires a level of skill that exercise machines do not. It's easier to make a mistake with a free weight: Your position may be off, or you could even drop it on yourself or someone else. The exercise machine locks you in the correct position, and there is very little risk of hitting yourself (or someone else) with a weight. True aficionados will argue that free weights give you a better workout because they engage a much larger muscle mass, but I think the workout that you get from well-chosen exercise machines can be just as good. I use exercise machines in my own workout.

Most people are amazed at the progress they make within a short of period of time. By the end of Cycle 1, you will probably see and feel a real difference in body strength and tone. Your muscles will feel tighter and more compact, and you'll be more confident and agile in your daily movements. In Cycle 2, you will see your muscles define themselves under your skin. Where there was once a smooth (or flabby) surface, there will be an attractive curve of muscle. In Cycle 3, you will continue to make great strides, putting your new muscle mass to work burning off any excess flab. This will take you from looking good to looking great!

Most people will achieve excellent results on the 6-Pack Prescription Workout. In fact, there are only two ways that you can fail. The first is if you are inconsistent. If you don't do the workout, you won't get its bene-fit. The second is if you do not exercise at a high enough level of inten-sity. If you breeze through your workouts, chances are, you will get very little out of them. You will just be wasting your time. You need to feel that you are working hard. (By that I don't mean writhing in pain with every lift: I don't want you to hurt yourself. If you feel sharp pain, stop whatever you're doing! It's a sign that you are not doing it correctly or that you have an injury.) By the time you are finishing your last repetitions on each set, you should be feeling that you are working to your maximum capacity. Anything less will not get you where you want to go. While I can give you some general guidelines on how to get the most out of your muscles, you alone can determine when you've really given it everything you've got.

In Cycle 1, you begin each day's workout with two warm-up sets to help you learn how to select your weights and use the equipment. If you are a novice at weight training, you may benefit by working out with a personal trainer for at least the first few weeks of the program. If you can't afford a personal trainer, most good gyms have a trainer on the floor who is available to answer questions. While they won't work with you one-on-one, they should be able to answer questions about a par-ticular machine or any problem that you may be having. If you are just joining a gym, most quality gyms will offer free orientation sessions dur-ing which the trainers will show you how to use the equipment.

In the pages that follow, I lay out the structure of the exercise plan, with specific instructions for each of the four cycles. In addition, you'll find a large how-to section with pictures of the exercises and clear in-structions for doing them. I've also included one workout chart for each

---

Work Out with a Friend

I find that it is great to have a workout partner with you at the gym. Find a friend and do the program together—or work out with your spouse. Many people find that having a partner whom they don't want to disappoint can motivate them to get to the gym, and that's half the battle.

cycle. These are the same kinds of charts that personal trainers use to track the progress of their clients. I find them quite helpful in keeping track of my workouts, and I think you will too. They are especially important for those of us (myself included) with busy lives and cluttered schedules. The charts free you from the duty of remembering your exercises, weights, settings, or even which day is up next. I've provided enough spaces to cover all twenty-four weeks of the program so that you can track your progress right in the book. If you'd rather download and print your own copy, I've posted copies of the charts on my Web site at www.bodyrxinfo.com. Following the charts is a frequently-asked-questions section. If you are new to exercising or uncomfortable about working out, I'd suggest going there first. There's even a primer on how to choose the right gym for you.

General Exercise Instructions

The 6-Pack Prescription Workout, like the food plan, is divided into four six-week cycles. While the general principles remain the same throughout the program, each cycle has its own goals for your physical development. The exercise system works synergistically with the food plan to make sure that both aspects of the program support the goal of better body composition.

CYCLE 1: GETTING STRONGER. Here you will lay down the basic strength and muscle coordination needed for a lifetime of better body composition.

CYCLE 2: GETTING SCULPTED. In these six weeks you will focus on gaining muscle size and definition. Here you will build lean muscle mass for both cosmetic effect and fat-burning potential.

CYCLE 3: BURNING FAT. Now it's time to concentrate the muscle you've built in the previous two cycles on the work of burning fat. You will already have seen remarkable changes in your body, but the big payoff is still to come. When you put the results of cycles 1 and 2 to work to maximize the rate of fat burning, you will go from looking good to looking great.

CYCLE 4: MAINTENANCE AND ENDURANCE. This is the maintenance program. Here you will build up your muscle endurance and develop the habits to keep the better body you have won.

You'll not only look and feel great, but you'll perform great. If you
play tennis, or golf, or enjoy shooting hoops on the weekend, you'll see
a real improvement in your game. Even if you aren't a sports enthusiast,
you will find that you have endurance to spare for everyday activities,
like climbing steps, or getting down on the floor and playing with your
kids, or making it through the workday without feeling exhausted.

The 6-Pack Prescription Workout operates on the principle of muscle exhaustion leading to muscle growth. Only by taking the muscle to
the limit of its capacity can you force it to adapt and grow. Your object is
to cause tiny injuries throughout the muscle. This controlled tissue
damage is *not* dangerous. It is the way our bodies were designed, as you
read in Chapter 6, "Body Rx: Exercise."

Each cycle exhausts the muscle in a particular way. Cycle 1 tears
down the fiber, leading to a rapid growth in strength. In this cycle you

The 6-Pack Prescription may be a six-month program, but it
doesn't mean that you should stop after six months. Ideally, when
you finish Cycle 4, you should start Cycle 1 all over again. Your
body will just keep getting better and better. Staying on the program will keep you in terrific shape for the rest of your life, and I
urge you to do so. If you're thrilled with your result after finishing
Cycle 4, however, and just want to maintain your new body, you
can go on a modified version of Cycle 4. Follow the Cycle 4 meal
plan, but follow only Weeks 1 and 2 of the Cycle 4 weight training
program (3 working sets, 12 repetitions each, with 1-minute rest
intervals.) Don't become complacent! Continue to exercise with
the right intensity, following the basic strategy of the program by
increasing the weight when the workout becomes too easy. And if
you ever get bored with doing the same regimen over and over, I
recommend that you start all over again with Cycle 1 for a change
of pace.

want to get as much out of your muscles as possible. Therefore, you will lift heavy weights for only a few repetitions. You will have a long rest period between sets of repetitions, allowing your muscles to recharge their store of molecular fuel—just like a flash recharging between photographs. In Cycle 2 you will decrease the rest period while increasing the number of repetitions, causing a more concentrated muscle exhaustion and rapid growth in muscle size, called hypertrophy. You will most likely be lifting a lighter weight (not by too much!), but the increased number of repetitions and shorter rest period will exhaust the muscle nonetheless. Cycle 3 shortens the rest period even further to maximize the fat-burning potential of your muscle mass. Once again, you will probably lift a lighter weight than you did at the end of Cycle 2, but your muscles will be working hard and burning up fuel at a furious pace. The various facets of Cycle 4 maintain your new muscle and add endurance for a lifetime of good health and a high performance lifestyle.

The exercise program has been designed as a four-day-a-week system. Do Day 1 first, Day 2 second, etc. Also, do the exercises for each day in the order they are listed. This ensures that you'll move the largest muscle groups first and gradually target the smaller ones for the most efficient workout possible. Each day's worth of exercise is repeated every seventh day, allowing for adequate recovery time. If you have limited time, the program can be done three days a week. Just carry the remaining day over into the next week. As long as you keep track of which set of exercises is next, you'll experience the same benefit. The charts that follow will be of great help in tracking where you are in the cycle.

How to Pick a Weight

Your working weight will vary according to the cycle.

FOR CYCLE 1: At the beginning of the cycle, for each exercise, start with a relatively light weight for you. If you can easily do 20 reps with a particular weight, then you know that you need to try a heavier weight. If it's really easy, try doubling the weight. If you drop down to 10 reps, then you need to keep increasing the weight (maybe by ¼) until you reach the point where you can do 6 reps with effort. But the weight should be heavy enough that by the third set, you have diffi-culty finishing the 6 reps: In fact, you may only do 4 to 5 reps. As you progress through the cycle your strength will increase. Once you can finish your 6 reps without struggling (and struggling means that you just barely make the last repetition), it's time to move up. (As a rule of thumb, increase your working load by about 10 percent at a time.) In the beginning, as you are gaining familiarity and coordination you may see rapid increases in strength. Soon these increases will level off and your progress, while just as real, will be less dramatic.

FOR CYCLE 2: At the beginning of the cycle you will select your work-ing weight by first trying lighter weights, then moving up incrementally until you find a weight that you can lift 8 to 10 times with effort. By the time you have reached your fourth or fifth set (I recommend 4 sets for big muscle groups, and 5 sets for small muscle groups), you should be working very hard and not be able to complete the set. In fact, you may only make it to 3 or 4 repetitions in your last set before finding your strength giving out. This feeling of exhaustion is different from the sen-sation you had in Cycle 1. While then you may have felt that the weight was just getting too hard to move, now you will feel as though you've just run out of gas. Once you have strengthened enough to get through the 10 lifts for each set, it's time to move up.

FOR CYCLE 3: As in the previous cycles, at the beginning of the cycle you will select your working weight by trying lighter weights, then moving up incrementally as it gets easier. You know that you've picked the right weight if, by the time you are doing your fifth or sixth set, you cannot complete the repetitions. The feeling of exhaustion is similar to that in Cycle 2. Once you can finish the set, you must move on to the next level to continue making gains.

FOR CYCLE 4: The same rules apply.

NOTE ABOUT ABDOMINAL EXERCISES: There is no set number of repetitions for abdominal exercises (pages 221 and 222). Simply do as many as you can in each set. Follow the instructions for the number of sets and the rest periods for each cycle.

CYCLE 1

6 weeks, 4 days a week

- 2 warm-up sets (light weight)
- 3 working sets
- 4–6 repetitions each set
- Move up in weight when you can complete the sixth repetition in the last set
- 3 minutes of rest between sets

CYCLE 2

6 weeks, 4 days a week

- Warm-up sets optional
- 4–5 working sets (4 for large muscle groups, 5 for small muscle groups)
- 8–10 repetitions each set
- Move up in weight when you can complete the tenth repetition in the last set (you may only get to 4 or so repetitions in the final set initially)
- 1½ minutes of rest between sets

CYCLE 3

6 weeks, 4 days a week

- Warm-up sets optional
- 5–6 working sets (5 for large muscle groups, 6 for small muscle groups)
- 6–12 repetitions each set
- Move up in weight when you can complete the twelfth repetition in the last set (you may only get to 4 or so repetitions in the final set initially)
- 1 minute of rest between sets

C Y C L E 4
6 weeks, divided into 2-week blocks, 4 days a week

W E E K S 1 – 2

- Warm-up sets optional

- 3 working sets

- 12 repetitions each set

- Move up in weight when you can complete the twelfth repetition in the last set

- 1 minute of rest between sets

W E E K S 3 – 4

- Warm-up sets optional

- 3 working sets

- 16 repetitions each set

- Move up in weight when you can complete the sixteenth repetition in the last set

- 1½ minutes of rest between each set

W E E K S 5 – 6

- Warm-up sets optional

- 3 working sets

- 20 repetitions each set

- Move up in weight when you can complete the twentieth repetition in the last set

- 2 minutes of rest between sets

DAY 1

Chest and Biceps

(1) Basic Machine Chest Press (*or* Alternate Chest Press)

(2) Incline Press (*or* Alternate Incline Press)

(3) Fly Maneuver (*or* Alternate Fly Maneuver)

(4) Dumbbell Curl

(5) Preacher Curl

DAY 2

Back and Triceps

(1) Lat Pull-Down

(2) Seated Row

(3) Seated Wide-Grip Row

(4) Tricep Push-Down

(5) Tricep Extension

DAY 3

Legs, Hamstrings, and Calves

(1) Leg Press

(2) Leg Extension

(3) Leg Curl

(4) Standing Calf Raise

(5) Donkey Calf Raise

DAY 4

Shoulders and Abs

(1) Basic Shoulder Press

(2) Seated Lateral Raise

(3) Rear Deltoid

(4) Forward Crunch

(5) Reverse Crunch

In Her Own Words

D E B K L I P P E R

I never had a problem with my weight until I went to college. My mom died of breast cancer during the third week of my freshman year. I know that it's common for people to gain weight during their first year away from home—there's even a name for it, the "Freshman 15"—but I was so stressed out, and eating so poorly, that I kept gaining. By the end of my junior year, I weighed 152, a lot for someone like me who's five-foot-five. It didn't bother me that much because everyone around me was gaining weight, too. That is, until I went on a vacation. When I got the pictures back, I was shocked by how bad I looked in a bathing suit. I wasn't just worried about my weight for cosmetic reasons. I knew that some types of breast cancer are related to estrogen levels, and I felt that carrying around all this excess weight meant that I was also carrying around a lot of extra estrogen. Since breast cancer runs in my family, I was determined to do whatever I could to reduce my risk. I was also motivated by the fact that heart disease runs on my father's side of the family, and being overweight is a risk factor for that disease. I decided it was time to take the weight off. I followed a typical low-calorie diet, and did

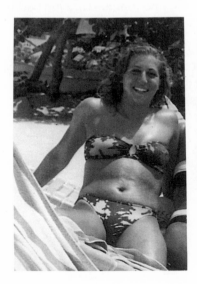
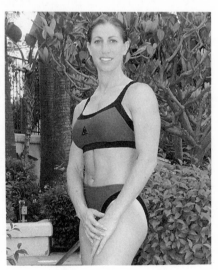

the standard exercise regimen of low weights, high reps, and aerobics. It took a year, but I managed to lose 15 pounds and got down to a size 8. Fine! The problem was, it was a real struggle staying there. Despite the fact that I was training hard and eating carefully, I still would put on weight easily. I was also concerned that at 242 mg/dl, my blood cholesterol levels were dangerously high given my family history for heart disease. For the next three years, with great effort, I maintained my size 8 body, but I was unable to lower my cholesterol. When I moved to California in 1996, I met Billy Carpenter (the nutritionist who helped design the 6-Pack System meal plan menus). He showed me why my low calorie diet wasn't working. I cut out some of the starchy carbs that had been the mainstay of my diet, and began to eat more protein, and within a short time, I was down to a size 6. Through Billy, I met Scott, who gave me the best advice of my life, that is, that I should work out the same way as a man works out, and forget about all this high-rep, low-weight nonsense. Scott put me on his nutrition and weight training program and the results were amazing. Within a year, I dropped four dress sizes (I'm now a size 2) and my cholesterol dropped to 187. I'm trimmer and leaner. The best part is, I'm no longer struggling to maintain my weight, in fact, I eat about 1,000 calories more than I did when I was a size 8! I feel great mentally and physically, and all the things that used to scare me about my family's health history no longer scare me because I know that I've taken control. By the way, I'm not a lady of leisure who lives at the gym. I work full time as a nurse in an outpatient clinic and am also going to graduate school to get a master's degree in nursing. My spare time is taken up by reading and writing papers. I still manage to get to the gym several times a week, and if I can do it, you can do it.

DAY 1 – EXERCISE 1
CHEST PRESS

Equipment: Basic Machine Press   **Muscle Group:** Whole Chest

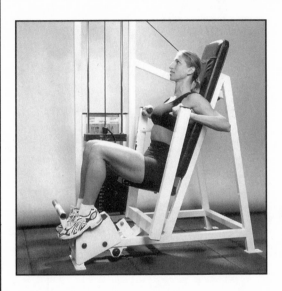
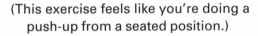
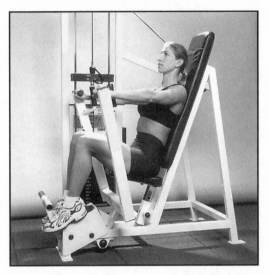

(This exercise feels like you're doing a push-up from a seated position.)

1. Sit comfortably in the chair.

2. Grip the handlebars on the arms of the chair. (Your hands should be at about shoulder height.)

3. Adjust your arms so that your elbows are raised to just below shoulder height.

4. If the machine has a foot pedal or bar (some will and some won't), depress it to bring the handlebars into position.

5. Push the handlebars away until your arms are fully extended.

6. Return the handlebars to your starting position.

DAY 1 - EXERCISE 1
ALTERNATE CHEST PRESS

Equipment: Free Weights   **Muscle Group:** Whole Chest

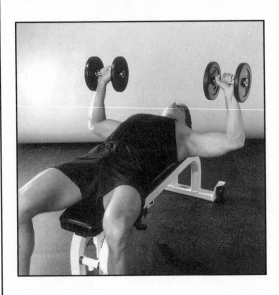 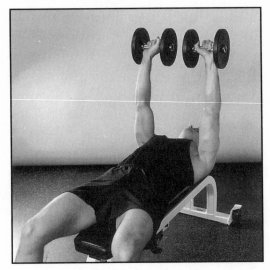

1. Lie on a flat bench with your feet firmly on the ground.

2. Hold the dumbbells parallel to your shoulders, in line with your chest and with your elbows making right angles.

3. Press the weights straight up until your arms are fully extended. Each weight should be directly above each shoulder.

4. Carefully return the weight to the starting position.

DAY 1 - EXERCISE 2
INCLINE PRESS

Equipment: Incline Press   **Muscle Group:** Upper Chest

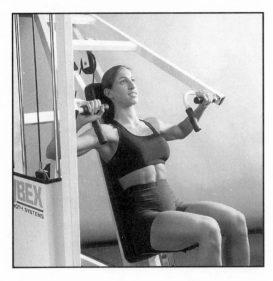 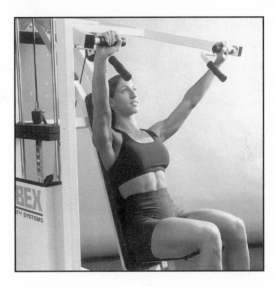

1. Sit down with your feet on the foot pedals. (If the machine doesn't have foot pedals, put your feet on the ground.)

2. Grip the handlebars (your hands should be at shoulder height) with your elbows out to the sides.

3. Push the handlebars up until your arms are fully extended.

4. Return the handlebars to your starting position.

DAY 1 - EXERCISE 2
ALTERNATE INCLINE PRESS

Equipment: Free Weights   **Muscle Group:** Upper Chest

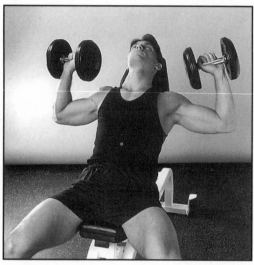 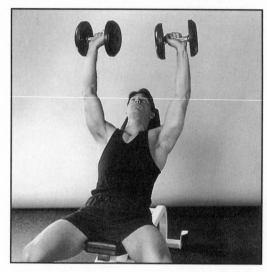

1. Lie on an inclined bench at a 45-degree angle with your feet on the floor.

2. Hold the dumbbells with your elbows bent at a 90-degree angle. Your shoulders should be in line with your collarbone, not hunched.

3. Press the weight straight up over your chest to the full extension of your elbows. Do not bring the weights together at the top of the movement. Keep your wrists straight or the weights will wobble.

4. Lower carefully to starting position.

DAY 1 - EXERCISE 3
FLY MANEUVER

Equipment: Chest Fly Machine   **Muscle Group:** Whole Chest

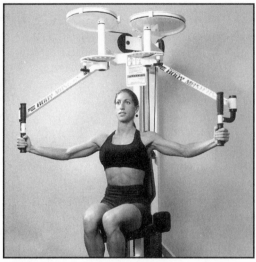 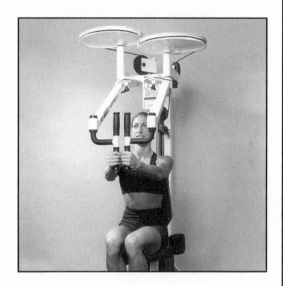

1. Adjust the seat height so that your arms are outstretched at a 90-degree angle to your body when you grasp the handlebars.

2. Sit down and extend your arms to grasp the handlebars with your elbows just slightly bent.˙

3. Keeping your arms extended, press your arms together until your fists meet.

4. Be careful not to bend your elbows further while performing the exercise.

5. Return to the starting position.

DAY 1 – EXERCISE 3
ALTERNATE FLY MANEUVER

Equipment: Free Weights   **Muscle Group:** Whole Chest

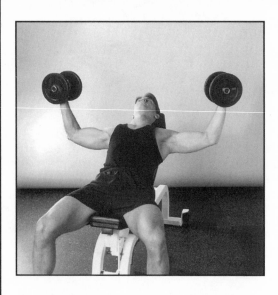 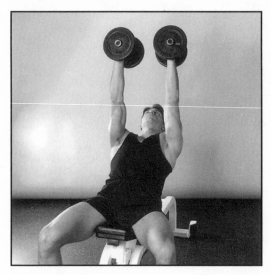

1. Lie on a bench inclined at about a 30-degree angle.

2. Grasping the dumbbells parallel to your body, extend your arms with your elbows slightly bent.

3. Raise the weights over your chest, extending your elbows, and bring the weights together at the top of the movement.

4. Carefully lower weights to starting position.

DAY 1 - EXERCISE 4
DUMBBELL CURL

Equipment: Free Weights   **Muscle Group:** Biceps

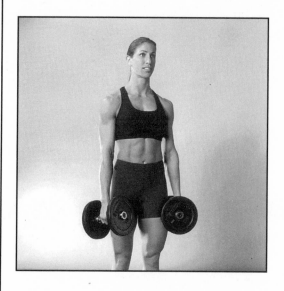 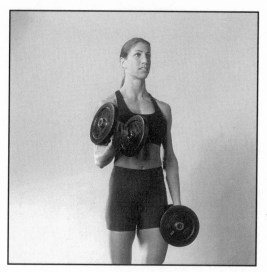

1. Stand straight-backed with your feet firmly placed shoulder-width apart.

2. Grip one dumbbell in each hand as you would a hammer with your wrists facing each other.

3. One arm at a time, raise the weight by bending at your elbow, holding the rest of your body immobile.

4. As you lift the weight past your thigh, turn your wrist so that your palm faces up. Bring the weight toward your shoulder.

5. Return to starting position.

6. Alternate arms. Note that you must complete your target number of repetitions *for each arm.*

DAY 1 - EXERCISE 5
PREACHER CURL

Equipment: Preacher curl bench and easy curl bar   **Muscle Group:** Biceps

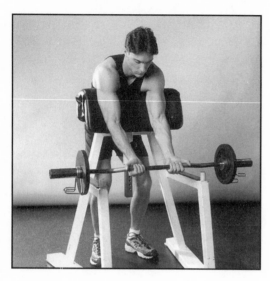 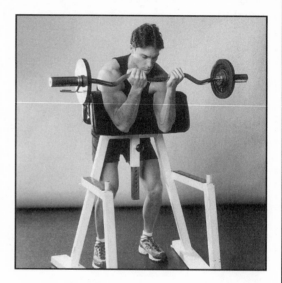

1. Stand at the bench with your knees slightly bent and your arms draped over the pad.

2. Grasp the barbell with an underhand grip and your wrists turned slightly inward.

3. Raise barbell to shoulders, keeping your upper arms pressed against the pad.

4. Lower weight carefully to starting position.

DAY 2 - EXERCISE 1
LAT PULL-DOWN

Equipment: Lat Pull-Down   **Muscle Group:** Upper Back

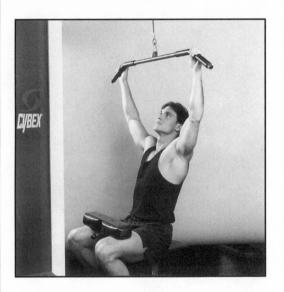 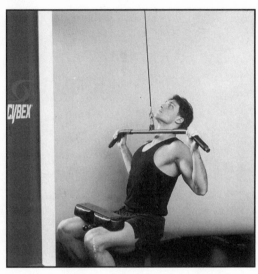

1. Sit down on the bench facing the pull-down bar with your legs firmly wedged beneath the padding.

2. Reach up to grasp the bar, holding it slightly wider than shoulder width.

3. Pull the bar down to your collarbone (slightly beneath your chin).

4. As you pull the bar, concentrate on keeping your shoulders low and your chest forward.

5. Return the bar to starting position.

Caution: Do not pull the bar behind your head. This position can cause acute injuries. (Yes, I know you'll see people doing this at the gym. They're wrong.)

DAY 2 - EXERCISE 2
SEATED ROW

Equipment: Cable Row with Small Handle Attachment   **Muscle Group:** Lower Back

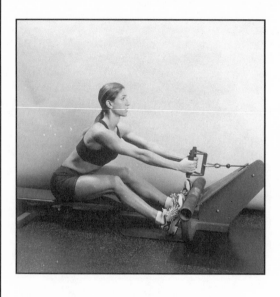 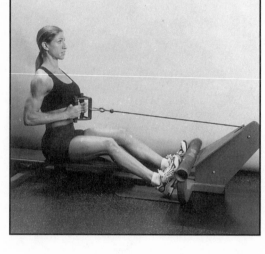

1. Start in a seated position with your feet pressed against the footpad and your knees slightly bent.

2. Reach forward to grab the handles on the cable. Bend from the waist and be careful not to hunch your back.

3. Sit back to an upright position while your arms smoothly pull the cables toward your lower abdomen.

4. Return to starting position.

DAY 2 - EXERCISE 3
SEATED WIDE–GRIP ROW

Equipment: Cable Row with Wide-Handle Attachment   **Muscle Group:** Whole Back

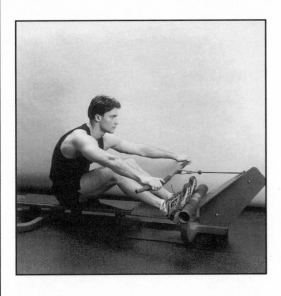 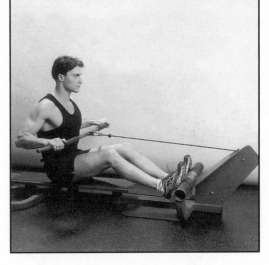

1. Start in a seated position with your feet pressed against the footpad and your knees slightly bent.

2. Reach forward to grab hold of the horizontal bar with your hands shoulder-width apart. Bend from the waist and try not to hunch your back.

3. Sit back to an upright position while your arms pull the bar toward your abdomen with your elbows flared outward at a right angle to your body.

4. Return to starting position.

DAY 2 - EXERCISE 4
TRICEPS PUSH-DOWN

Equipment: Push-Down Station   **Muscle Group:** Triceps

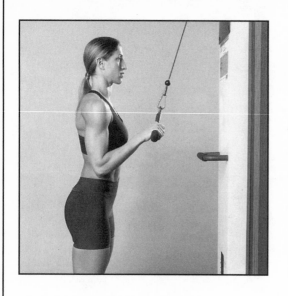 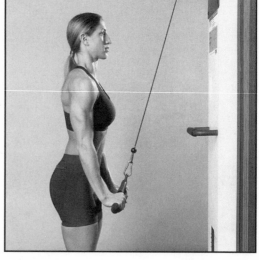

1. Start in a standing position.

2. Grip the bar with your hands at hip width. Keep your elbows slightly flexed and close to your body.

3. Push the bar straight down as far as you can.

4. Return to starting position slowly, remaining under control. Don't allow your elbows to move outward.

DAY 2 - EXERCISE 5
TRICEPS EXTENSION

Equipment: Free Weights   **Muscle Group:** Triceps

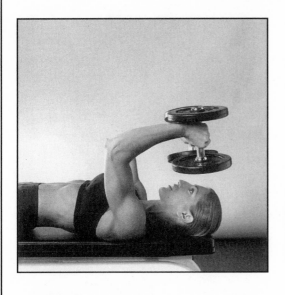 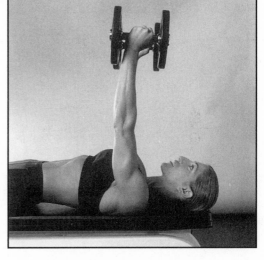

1. Lie flat on a bench.

2. With dumbbells in your hands, bend your arms into an L shape with the weights hovering just over your forehead.

3. Extend your arms straight up, bending only at the elbows, until your arms are fully extended.

4. Carefully lower the weights to starting position.

   Caution: Don't drop the weights on your face. No kidding. It hurts. If you don't feel confident doing this, have someone spot you.

A Note for Day 3: *Legs*

Your legs (hamstrings, calves, quadriceps, and buttocks) are by far the strongest muscles in your body. After all, they support your weight all day, every day! As a result, you will find that you can move an enormous amount of weight with your legs. Don't be surprised if the weights you use are much higher than those for your upper body.

DAY 3 - EXERCISE 1
LEG PRESS

Equipment: Leg Press **Muscle Group:** Whole Leg (Quadriceps, Hamstrings, and Calves)

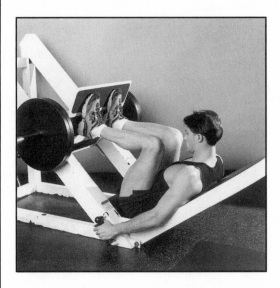 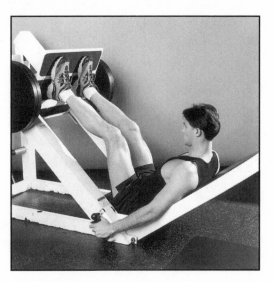

1. Sit in the chair with the backrest at a 30–45-degree angle from the floor. Make sure your back is fully pressed against the backrest and that your hips are firmly seated. Your body should be in a right angle, bent at the hip.

2. Raise your legs up so that your toes are an inch or two below the edge of the plate. Keep your feet shoulder-width apart, pointed straight ahead.

3. Press up to extend the machine, and grasp the handles at your hips to rotate the weight catch out of the way. Use the handles to brace your body as you complete the exercise.

4. Lower the weight until your knees are flexed and your hips are just about to rotate out of the firmly seated position. Your knees will be at a 45-degree angle. This is the starting position.

5. Push up against the plate until your knees are fully extended, but not locked. If you feel pain in your knees, readjust your feet. They could be too high on the plate or too low.

6. Return to starting position.

7. After you finish your set, fully extend the machine and rotate the weight catches back into place.

DAY 3 - EXERCISE 2
LEG EXTENSION

Equipment: Leg-Extension   **Muscle Group:** Quadriceps

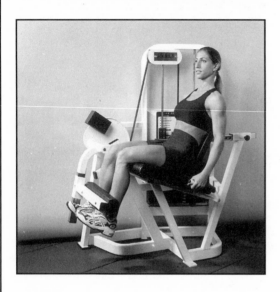 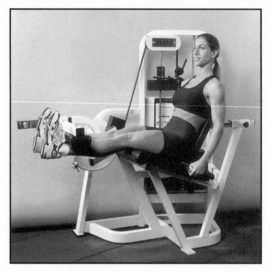

1. Sit on the chair with your back straight.

2. Place your feet under the ankle pad with your toes pointed straight ahead. The pad should rest just above your ankle joint. Adjust as necessary.

3. Lift your legs up until your knees are fully extended.

4. *Slowly* return to starting position.

DAY 3 - EXERCISE 3
LEG CURL

Equipment: Leg Curl   **Muscle Group:** Hamstrings

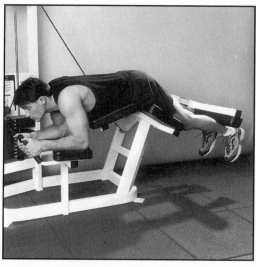

1. Lie down on your stomach.

2. Hold on to the hand grips for stability.

3. Make sure the ankle pad is placed right above your ankles, behind your Achilles tendon.

4. Bring your legs up toward your buttocks as far as you can.

5. Return to starting position.

   Caution: Avoid leg curl machines that have flat benches: they can hurt your back.

DAY 3 – EXERCISE 4
STANDING CALF RAISE

Equipment: Standing Calf Raise   **Muscle Group:** Calves

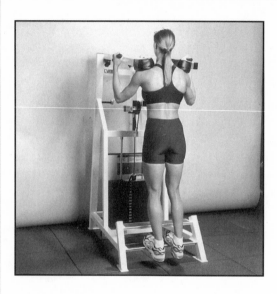
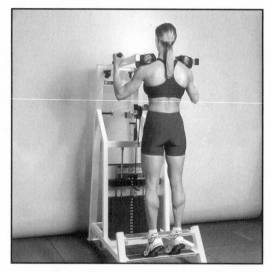

1. Grip the handrails. Stand straight. Place the balls of your feet on the edge of the step plate.

2. Place the weight pad on your shoulders.

3. Rise up on the balls of your feet as high as you can, being careful to keep your feet parallel.

4. Return to starting position.

DAY 3 - EXERCISE 5
DONKEY CALF RAISE

Equipment: Donkey Calf Raise   **Muscle Group:** Calves

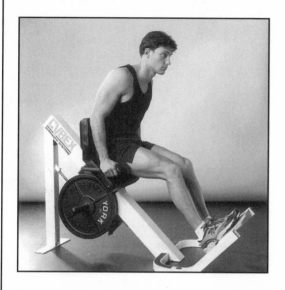 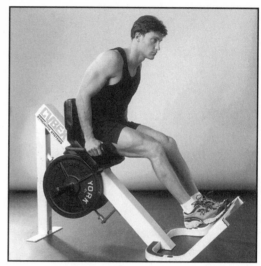

1. Sit on the chair with your upper body leaning slightly forward. Rest the balls of your feet against the foot plate and push back until your knees are only slightly bent. Grip the handrails for support. This is the starting position.

2. Push up on the balls of your feet (just as you did with the Standing Calf Raise).

3. Return to starting position.

DAY 4 – EXERCISE 1
BASIC SHOULDER PRESS

Equipment: Shoulder Press   **Muscle Group:** Shoulders

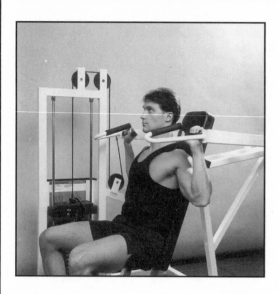
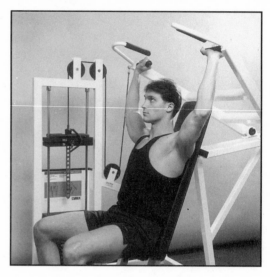

1. Grab the handrails with your hands facing forward and your elbows flared outward. Adjust the seat so that your elbows are bent into a right angle.

2. Push up to full extension.

3. Return to starting position.

DAY 4 - EXERCISE 2
SEATED LATERAL RAISE

Equipment: Dumbbells   **Muscle Group:** Deltoids (Shoulder Caps)

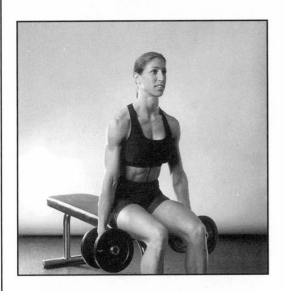 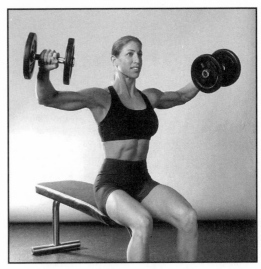

1. Sit upright on a bench with a dumb-bell in each hand.

2. Start with your arms at your sides and your wrists straight.

3. Lift the weights up to around shoulder height, rotating from your shoulder joint. Think of the dumbbell as a pitcher of water, so as you raise your arms, you are pouring the water and your thumb turns downward. Your elbows are kept slightly bent.

4. Return to starting position.

DAY 4 - EXERCISE 3
REAR DELTOIDS

Equipment: Chest Fly Machine   **Muscle Group:** Rear Deltoids

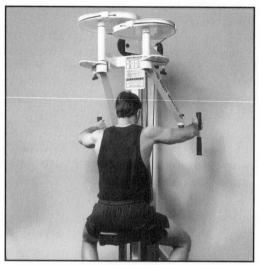 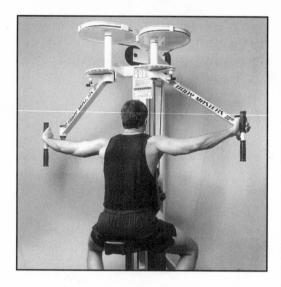

1. Rotate the arms of the fly machine fully inward and lock in position.

2. Sit facing the machine and adjust the seat so that your arms are straight out in front of you, at a right angle to your body.

3. Grasp the handles and pull apart until your arms are fully open.

4. Slowly return to starting position.

DAY 4 - EXERCISE 4
FORWARD CRUNCH

Equipment: Bench   **Muscle Group:** Abdominals

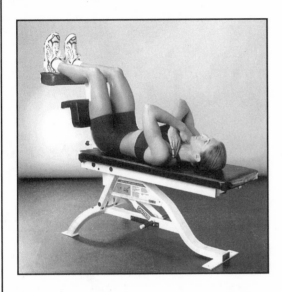 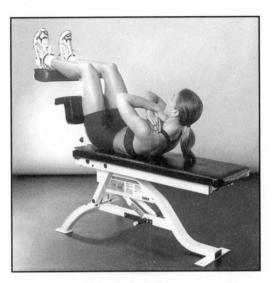

1. Lie down with your arms crossed on your chest.

2. Place your feet on top of the footrest (not underneath it!). You want your legs to be in a free-floating position, not a fixed position. (Remember all those sit-ups you did in gym class with someone sitting on your feet? They were a waste of time.)

3. Lift your trunk as far off the surface as you can toward your hips. Imagine that you are trying to bring your rib cage and hips together. Your range of motion will be very limited. This is a tough exercise.

4. Return to starting position.

*Note: Do not add resistance to this exercise. Your body weight is enough. In all four cycles, simply do as many reps as you are able in each set. Follow the instructions for the number of sets and the rest periods for each cycle.

DAY 4 - EXERCISE 5
REVERSE CRUNCH

Equipment: Bench   **Muscle Group:** Abdominals

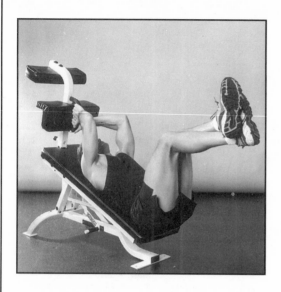
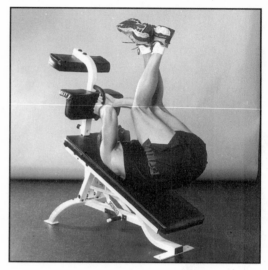

1. Lie flat on the floor or on a bench. Fix your legs at a 90-degree angle with your ankles crossed.

2. Lift the small of your back off the mat toward your breastbone. Once again, imagine that you are trying to bring your rib cage and hips together, only this time from the other direction. You will be able to lift only a few inches. Do not swing your legs. This will only add momentum and will thereby defeat the purpose of the exercise.

3. Return to starting position.

   *Note: Do not add resistance to this exercise. Your body is enough. In all four cycles, simply do as many reps as you are able in each set.

CYCLE 1
Getting Stronger

HOW TO USE THESE CHARTS

- Record your seat position for each exercise (if necessary).

- Record the weight you used in your last set in the top part of each box.

- Record the number of repetitions you achieved on your last set in the bottom of each box.

- You will make one circuit through the 4 charts each week, recording that information in the Week 1 column. The next week, move one column over, and so on until the cycle is complete.

CYCLE INSTRUCTIONS

- 2 warm-up sets (40% of your working load weight).

- 3 working sets.

- 4–6 repetitions each set.

- You should not be able to finish 6 repetitions on the final set. If you do, advance weight by 10%.

- 3 minutes of rest between sets.

- For abs, since you don't use any weights, do repetitions of each exercise until exhaustion. Repeat for 3 sets. Record in the box the number of reps you achieved in your last set.

HOW TO PICK YOUR WEIGHT

At the beginning of the cycle, for each exercise, start with a relatively light weight for you. If you can easily do 20 reps with a particular weight, then you know that you need to try a heavier weight. Try doubling the weight. If you drop down to 10 reps, then you need to keep increasing the weight (maybe by ¼) until you reach the point where you can do six reps with effort. The weight should be heavy enough that by the third set, you can only do 4–5 reps. Once you can finish your 6 reps without struggling, it's time to move up. (As a rule of thumb, increase your working load by about 10% at a time.)

DAY 1

Chest and Biceps

Exercise	Seat	Week 1	Week 2	Week 3	Week 4	Week 5	Week 6
Chest Press							
Incline Press							
Fly Maneuver							
Dumbbell Curl							
Preacher Curl							

CYCLE 1 INSTRUCTIONS

- 2 warm-up sets (40% of your working load weight).
- 3 working sets.
- 4–6 repetitions each set.

- You should not be able to finish 6 repetitions on the final set. If you do, advance weight by 10%.
- 3 minutes of rest between sets.

DAY 2

Back and Triceps

Exercise	Seat	Week 1	Week 2	Week 3	Week 4	Week 5	Week 6
Lat Pull-Down							
Seated Row							
Wide-Grip Row							
Triceps Push-Down							
Triceps Extension							

CYCLE 1 INSTRUCTIONS

- 2 warm-up sets (40% of your working load weight).
- 3 working sets.
- 4–6 repetitions each set.

- You should not be able to finish 6 repetitions on the final set. If you do, advance weight by 10%.
- 3 minutes of rest between sets.

DAY 3

Legs, Hamstrings, and Calves

Exercise	Seat	Week 1	Week 2	Week 3	Week 4	Week 5	Week 6
Leg Press							
Leg Extension							
Leg Curl							
Standing Calf-Raise							
Donkey Calf-Raise							

CYCLE 1 INSTRUCTIONS

- 2 warm-up sets (40% of your working load weight).
- 3 working sets.
- 4–6 repetitions each set.
- You should not be able to finish 6 repetitions on the final set. If you do, advance weight by 10%.
- 3 minutes of rest between sets.

DAY 4

Shoulders and Abs

Exercise	Seat	Week 1	Week 2	Week 3	Week 4	Week 5	Week 6
Shoulder Press							
Seated Lat Raise							
Rear Deltoid							
Forward Crunch (reps only)							
Reverse Crunch (reps only)							

CYCLE 1 INSTRUCTIONS

- 2 warm-up sets (40% of your working load weight).
- 3 working sets.
- 4–6 repetitions each set.
- You should not be able to finish 6 repetitions on the final set. If you do, advance weight by 10%.
- 3 minutes of rest between sets.
- For abs, since you don't use any weights, do repetitions of each exercise until exhaustion. Repeat 3 sets. Record in the box the number of reps you achieved in your last set.

CYCLE 2
Getting Sculpted

HOW TO USE THESE CHARTS

- Record your seat position for each exercise.

- Record the weight you used in your last set in the top part of each box.

- Record the number of repetitions you achieved on your last set in the bottom of each box.

- You will make one circuit through the 4 charts each week, recording that information in the Week 1 column. The next week, move one column over, and so on until the cycle is complete.

CYCLE INSTRUCTIONS

- Warm-up sets optional.

- 4–5 working sets.

- 8–10 repetitions each set.

- You should not be able to finish 10 repetitions on the final set. If you do, advance weight by 10%.

- No more than 1½ minutes of rest between sets.

- For abs, since you don't use any weights, do repetitions of each exercise until exhaustion. Repeat for 4 sets. Record in the box the number of reps you achieved in your last set.

HOW TO PICK YOUR WEIGHT

At the beginning of the cycle you will select your working weight by first trying lighter weights and moving up incrementally until you find a weight that you can lift 8–10 times with effort. By the time you reach your fourth or fifth set (4 sets recommended for large muscle groups, 5 sets for small muscle groups), you should be working very hard and should not be able to complete the set. Once you have strengthened enough to get through the 10 lifts for each set, it's time to move up.

DAY 1

Chest and Biceps

Exercise	Seat	Week 1	Week 2	Week 3	Week 4	Week 5	Week 6
Chest Press							
Incline Press							
Fly Maneuver							
Dumbbell Curl							
Preacher Curl							

CYCLE 2 INSTRUCTIONS

- Warm-up sets optional.
- 4–5 working sets.
- 8–10 repetitions each set.

- You should not be able to finish 10 repetitions on the final set. If you do, advance weight by 10%.
- No more than 1½ minutes of rest between sets.

DAY 2

Back and Triceps

Exercise	Seat	Week 1	Week 2	Week 3	Week 4	Week 5	Week 6
Lat Pull-Down							
Seated Row							
Wide-Grip Row							
Triceps Push-Down							
Triceps Extension							

CYCLE 2 INSTRUCTIONS

- Warm-up sets optional.
- 4–5 working sets.
- 8–10 repetitions each set.

- You should not be able to finish 10 repetitions on the final set. If you do, advance weight by 10%.
- No more than 1½ minutes of rest between sets.

DAY 3

Legs, Hamstrings, and Calves

Exercise	Seat	Week 1	Week 2	Week 3	Week 4	Week 5	Week 6
Leg Press							
Leg Extension							
Leg Curl							
Standing Calf-Raise							
Donkey Calf-Raise							

CYCLE 2 INSTRUCTIONS

- Warm-up sets optional.
- 4–5 working sets.
- 8–10 repetitions each set.

- You should not be able to finish 10 repetitions on the final set. If you do, advance weight by 10%.
- No more than 1½ minutes of rest between sets.

DAY 4

Shoulders and Abs

Exercise	Seat	Week 1	Week 2	Week 3	Week 4	Week 5	Week 6
Shoulder Press							
Seated Lat Raise							
Rear Deltoid							
Forward Crunch (reps only)							
Reverse Crunch (reps only)							

CYCLE 2 INSTRUCTIONS

- Warm-up sets optional.
- 4–5 working sets.
- 8–10 repetitions each set.
- You should not be able to finish 10 repetitions on the final set. If you do, advance weight by 10%.
- No more than 1½ minutes of rest between sets.
- For abs, since you don't use any weights, do repetitions of each exercise until exhaustion. Repeat for 4 sets. Record in the box the number of reps you achieved in your last set.

CYCLE 3
Burning Fat

HOW TO USE THESE CHARTS

- Record your seat position for each exercise.

- Record the weight you used in your last set in the top part of each box.

- Record the number of repetitions you achieved on your last set in the bottom of each box.

- You will make one circuit through the 4 charts each week, recording that information in the Week 1 column. The next week, move one column over, and so on until the cycle is complete.

CYCLE INSTRUCTIONS

- Warm-up sets optional.

- 5–6 working sets.

- 6–12 repetitions each set.

- You should not be able to finish 12 repetitions on the final set. If you do, advance weight by 10%.

- Rest for 60 seconds between sets.

- For abs, since you don't use any weights, do repetitions of each exercise until exhaustion. Repeat for 5 sets. Record in the box the number of reps you achieved in your last set.

HOW TO PICK YOUR WEIGHT

Similar to the previous cycles, at the beginning of the cycle you will select your working weight by trying lighter weights and moving up incrementally as it gets easier. You will know that you've picked the right weight if by the time you are doing your fifth or sixth set, you cannot complete the repetitions. Once you can finish the set, you must move on to the next level to continue making gains.

DAY 1

Chest and Biceps

Exercise	Seat	Week 1	Week 2	Week 3	Week 4	Week 5	Week 6
Chest Press							
Incline Press							
Fly Maneuver							
Dumbbell Curl							
Preacher Curl							

CYCLE 3 INSTRUCTIONS

- Warm-up sets optional.
- 5–6 working sets.
- 6–12 repetitions each set.

- You should not be able to finish 12 repetitions on the final set. If you do, advance weight by 10%.
- Rest for 60 seconds between sets.

DAY 2

Back and Triceps

Exercise	Seat	Week 1	Week 2	Week 3	Week 4	Week 5	Week 6
Lat Pull-Down							
Seated Row							
Wide-Grip Row							
Triceps Push-Down							
Triceps Extension							

CYCLE 3 INSTRUCTIONS

- Warm-up sets optional.
- 5–6 working sets.
- 6–12 repetitions each set.
- You should not be able to finish 12 repetitions on the final set. If you do, advance weight by 10%.
- Rest for 60 seconds between sets.

DAY 3

Legs, Hamstrings, and Calves

Exercise	Seat	Week 1	Week 2	Week 3	Week 4	Week 5	Week 6
Leg Press							
Leg Extension							
Leg Curl							
Standing Calf-Raise							
Donkey Calf-Raise							

CYCLE 3 INSTRUCTIONS

- Warm-up sets optional.
- 5–6 working sets.
- 6–12 repetitions each set.

- You should not be able to finish 12 repetitions on the final set. If you do, advance weight by 10%.
- Rest for 60 seconds between sets.

DAY 4

Shoulders and Abs

Exercise	Seat	Week 1	Week 2	Week 3	Week 4	Week 5	Week 6
Shoulder Press							
Seated Lat Raise							
Rear Deltoid							
Forward Crunch (reps only)							
Reverse Crunch (reps only)							

CYCLE 3 INSTRUCTIONS

- Warm-up sets optional.
- 5–6 working sets.
- 6–12 repetitions each set.
- You should not be able to finish 10 repetitions on the final set. If you do, advance weight by 10%.
- Rest for 60 seconds between sets.
- For abs, since you don't use any weights, do repetitions of each exercise until exhaustion. Repeat for 5 sets. Record in the box the number of reps you achieved in your last set .

CYCLE 4
Maintenance and Endurance

HOW TO USE THESE CHARTS

- Record your seat position for each exercise (if necessary).

- Record the weight you used in your last set in the top part of each box.

- Record the number of repetitions you achieved on your last set in the bottom of each box.

- You will make one circuit through the 4 charts each week, recording that information in the Week 1 column. The next week, move one column over, and so on until the cycle is complete.

CYCLE INSTRUCTIONS

WEEKS 1 – 2

- Warm-up sets optional.
- 3 working sets.
- 12 repetitions each set.
- Rest for 1 minute between sets.

WEEKS 3 – 4

- Warm-up sets optional.
- 3 working sets.
- 16 repetitions each set.
- Rest for 1½ minutes between sets.

WEEKS 5 – 6

- Warm-up sets optional.
- 3 working sets.
- 20 repetitions each set.
- Rest for 2 minutes between sets.

HOW TO PICK YOUR WEIGHT

The same rules apply as in earlier cycles.

DAY 1

Chest and Biceps

Exercise	Seat	Week 1	Week 2	Week 3	Week 4	Week 5	Week 6
Chest Press							
Incline Press							
Fly Maneuver							
Dumbbell Curl							
Preacher Curl							

CYCLE 4 INSTRUCTIONS

WEEKS 1–2

- Warm-up sets optional.
- 3 working sets.
- 12 repetitions each set.
- Rest for 1 minute between sets.

WEEKS 3–4

- Warm-up sets optional.
- 3 working sets.
- 16 repetitions each set.
- Rest for 1½ minutes between sets.

WEEKS 5–6

- Warm-up sets optional.
- 3 working sets.
- 20 repetitions each set.
- Rest for 2 minutes between sets.

DAY 2

Back and Triceps

Exercise	Seat	Week 1	Week 2	Week 3	Week 4	Week 5	Week 6
Lat Pull-Down							
Seated Row							
Wide-Grip Row							
Triceps Push-Down							
Triceps Extension							

CYCLE 4 INSTRUCTIONS

WEEKS 1–2

- Warm-up sets optional.
- 3 working sets.
- 12 repetitions each set.
- Rest for 1 minute between sets.

WEEKS 3–4

- Warm-up sets optional.
- 3 working sets.
- 16 repetitions each set.
- Rest for 1½ minutes between sets.

WEEKS 5–6

- Warm-up sets optional.
- 3 working sets.
- 20 repetitions each set.
- Rest for 2 minutes between sets.

DAY 3

Legs, Hamstrings, and Calves

Exercise	Seat	Week 1	Week 2	Week 3	Week 4	Week 5	Week 6
Leg Press							
Leg Extension							
Leg Curl							
Standing Calf-Raise							
Donkey Calf-Raise							

CYCLE 4 INSTRUCTIONS

WEEKS 1–2
- Warm-up sets optional.
- 3 working sets.
- 12 repetitions each set.
- Rest for 1 minute between sets.

WEEKS 3–4
- Warm-up sets optional.
- 3 working sets.
- 16 repetitions each set.
- Rest for 1½ minutes between sets.

WEEKS 5–6
- Warm-up sets optional.
- 3 working sets.
- 20 repetitions each set.
- Rest for 2 minutes between sets.

DAY 4

Shoulders and Abs

Exercise	Seat	Week 1	Week 2	Week 3	Week 4	Week 5	Week 6
Shoulder Press							
Seated Lat Raise							
Rear Deltoid							
Forward Crunch (reps only)							
Reverse Crunch (reps only)							

CYCLE 4 INSTRUCTIONS

WEEKS 1–2
- Warm-up sets optional.
- 3 working sets.
- 12 repetitions each set.
- Rest for 1 minute between sets.

WEEKS 3–4
- Warm-up sets optional.
- 3 working sets.
- 16 repetitions each set.
- Rest for 1½ minutes between sets.

WEEKS 5–6
- Warm-up sets optional.
- 3 working sets.
- 20 repetitions each set.
- Rest for 2 minutes between sets.

Frequently Asked Questions

How fast will I make progress?

Most people will make rapid progress early in Cycle 1, the strength-building phase, especially if they are new to weight training. Here women have a decided advantage over men: Due to hormonal differences, women actually make faster progress at this stage than men! For the first three weeks, many of you will find that you are able to steadily increase your weight each week. In fact, it's possible that you will double or even triple the amount of weight you can lift within a short period of time. In order to make these gains, however, you will have to keep increasing your weight as soon as you are ready. When you can do 3 sets of the 6 repetitions without struggling, it's time to move on. (See "How to Pick Your Weight.") However, you will eventually plateau and your gains will inevitably slow down within a few weeks. Don't be discouraged. You will still be making improvements, albeit in a less dramatic fashion.

More experienced weight lifters will not make as rapid progress as novices; that's because they are closer to their peak performance. When I start a strength-training program, I'm thrilled if I can make a 10-to-15-percent improvement over six weeks. When you stop making quick progress, all it means is that you are getting stronger.

It's not essential to make constant gains every week or so. Small but consistent gains will add up to a big win.

I'm self-conscious about my body and hate the thought of working out at a gym. What are my alternatives?

Your question tells me that you haven't walked into a gym lately. Gyms today are filled with people of all ages, in all levels of fitness, from all walks of life. And if you walk into the gym armed with your program, you will be better prepared for your workout than most of the people whom you will encounter. Working with a personal trainer for the first few weeks may be all it takes to make you feel confident. In addition, there are many different kinds of gyms. For example, you may feel more comfortable at a smaller gym than a larger one. Or your local Y may attract a less intimidating crowd than the commercial gym. Be sure to check out all your options; I'm sure you'll find the right fit.

Is it normal to feel sore after working out?

It's not only normal, but necessary. In fact, if you don't feel sore after your workout, it means that you are not working out hard enough. Remember, the way you make muscle grow is to injure it, and when muscle is injured, it becomes inflamed, and that's why you hurt. It takes about 24 to 36 hours for the inflammation to reach its peak. Post-workout pain, also known as delayed onset muscle soreness (DOMS), is a good sign, because it means that you are giving it your all. If you're in a lot of discomfort, do as I do: Take ibuprofen. However, I've designed the program so that you are not exercising your whole body every day. You won't be sore in more than one area at a time. And anyway, I think you'll find the soreness to be rather minor.

Do I have to warm up before working out?
Will stretching first prevent injuries?

Personally, I don't do warm-ups and I never stretch. I do recommend two warm-up sets for Cycle 1, primarily to get you used to exercises. Warm-ups are not necessary: Your muscles will warm up after the first few repetitions of any exercise. If you want to warm up before lifting, you can do 5 to 10 minutes on a treadmill or exercise bike, but no more. There is absolutely no evidence that stretching before lifting prevents injuries. If you like to stretch, and it makes you feel good, go ahead and do it. Just don't be overzealous about it. Stretching too vigorously can hurt your joints.

Should women do the same exercises as men?

Yes! One of the prevailing myths is that women should be doing something different at the gym than men. Many trainers are guilty of bringing a woman into the gym, adjusting the machine to the lowest weight, and then having the woman do endless numbers of repetitions. The whole exercise adds up to a complete waste of time. There is absolutely no evidence that any parameter of strength training should be substantially modified between men and women. On an absolute scale, women may lift lighter weights because men are generally stronger, especially in the upper body, but women's lower body strength is often comparable to men. Women need to approach strength training with an open mind. They need to determine what weight they are capable of lifting—not what they think they can lift.

Many women are surprised by their own strength. There are several common exercises (for example, squats) that I see women doing in the gym all the time. I'm not a fan of these movements because they can develop women in ways that many feel are unflattering. Stick to the exercises in this program, no matter if you are a man or a woman, to sculpt your body most attractively.

Should teenagers do weight training?

I know that some so-called experts say that teenagers shouldn't lift weights, but there's no scientific basis to this. I've been weight training since I was 11, and I think it makes a great deal of sense for kids to develop muscle strength. This is particularly true for teenage girls, who are often obsessed about their weight. In addition, teenagers engage in all kinds of vigorous, even dangerous sports, and a major cause of injury is due to poorly trained muscles! Many gyms, however, do not want teenagers working out without adult supervision. The rationale is that teenagers may not always exercise the best judgment and may be more prone to do risky things. I'm not sure whether or not this is true—I've seen some adults do some pretty stupid things at the gym—but to be on the safe side, if a teenager wants to do weight training, he or she should take a class or work with a trainer. Some enlightened gyms have special classes and programs for teenagers, and some high schools are even offering resistance-training classes instead of the usual gym classes. I would not advise teenagers to work out with free weights at home.

Why don't you recommend exercising the same muscle groups every day?

Keep in mind that it's not the actual workout that grows muscle; all the adaptive growth occurs during recovery. If you constantly overstimulate a muscle, you don't give it adequate time to recover, and it won't grow properly and it won't heal. In fact, overtraining causes overuse injuries, which can cause a great deal of unnecessary pain and suffering and actually keep you out of the gym.

I've never joined a gym before. How do I pick a good one?

There are many different types of gyms designed to appeal to different types of people and different budgets. Some gyms are for serious body builders; others are for recreational exercises; some are luxurious (with really nice locker rooms and TVs and CD players on every treadmill), while others are more basic. Before joining a gym, be sure to take a tour of the facility. Be especially sure that you feel comfortable in the environment there. If a gym makes you uneasy or just doesn't feel "right" for you, don't join. If you do, you probably won't go. Here are some other things to look for:

- A good gym should offer a variety of new, well-maintained equipment. Broken equipment should be repaired quickly. The gym should look clean. Ask the manager what the policy is about repairing exercise equipment. A good facility usually has a service that comes in fairly frequently to update and fix the equipment.

- Many gyms offer flexible memberships that allow members to pay by the day, week, month or even year. Some gyms even have initiation fees. Be sure that you understand your financial commitment before signing up. If you are unsure about a gym, try to join for as short a time as possible to see if you like it.

- Check out traffic patterns. If you are only able to use the gym during its peak times, be sure that it's not so overcrowded that you have to wait a long time before you can use a piece of equipment. Also, if you tend to use the gym during peak hours, make sure that there's room for your car in the parking lot, if that's an issue. Moreover, you are much more likely to attend a gym that's easy to get to. So, don't join the "perfect" gym if it's a pain to get to.

I enjoy my aerobics class. Do I have to give it up while I'm doing weight training?

If you want to do aerobics along with weight training, you can, as long as you don't overdo it. I don't recommend more than 20 to 30 minutes of aerobics every other day. In fact, adding an aerobic workout in Cycle 3 can give some extra oomph to your fat burning, but it's certainly not necessary. My only problem with aerobics is that it is no substitute for strength training, and given a choice between working with weights or aerobics, I would always pick weight training. If you have limited time for exercise, which most of us do, you are better off trying to focus 100 percent of your time on weight training than trying to mix the two. If you have the time and it is important to you, you can add an aerobic component to your workout.

Why shouldn't people work out at home?

I'm very skeptical of programs that promise that you can do a complete workout at home. First of all, few people have the correct equipment in their home gyms. In order to get the benefits of this program, you need to be lifting heavy weights on safe equipment. That said, if you have a complete set of dumbbells and a bench at home, you can do most of the upper body exercises, but be careful! If you are an experienced lifter, go ahead and do what you can at home. If, however, you are a novice, I'd recommend that you either go to the gym or work at home under some experienced supervision. However, unless you have a complete home gym, you will find it impossible to give your lower body a sufficiently vigorous workout.

There is another reason why I discourage working out at home. Few people have the discipline to exercise on a regular basis by themselves. There are too many distractions at home, and too many reasons not to exercise. I think that the gym is an environment that is more conducive to exercise. There is also a camaraderie at a gym that you don't experience working out by yourself at home.

What if I fall off the program for a while?

Things can happen in life (like a divorce, a job change, a death in the family) that can temporarily derail you, but all is not lost. Once you have gained a certain amount of muscle conditioning, when you begin to train again, returning to that point is a lot easier than getting there in the first place. The phenomenon is called muscle memory. Follow the program from the beginning, and you should be able to resume your level of fitness within a short period of time.

I would like to make one point: People tend to stop coming to the gym during times of acute stress. This is a mistake. Working out is a wonderful stress reliever, and I believe that it can help you better navigate through troubled times. What good are you to others if you do not maintain your own health?

There is a leg exercise that is not on your list that works well for me. If I follow your program, do I have to stop doing it?

Although the 6-Pack Prescription workout plan is comprehensive, it doesn't include every exercise machine at the gym. If there is an exercise that you particularly enjoy, you can still do it, with the following caveats. First, whatever exercise you do, follow the principles of the program. Do the exercise with the correct intensity, and be sure that you are challenging yourself sufficiently. That means that you should follow my recommended set, repetition, and rest interval principles set forth earlier in this book. Second, if you add an additional exercise to your workout, be sure that you aren't overworking a particular muscle group on the same day. Drop one of the other exercises, or do the exercise you like a few days later.

Can I combine two exercise regimens (like Day 1 and Day 2) on the same day?

You can if you want, as long as you don't tire out. There is a risk that you will run out of steam before you're through with the second workout. If possible, try to do one in the morning and one in the afternoon or evening to give your body time to recharge.

Part III

Dr. Connelly's Intensive Care
for Special Situations

8

Body R_x: Supplements

The combination of the right nutrition and the right work will help

you achieve your goal of a strong, healthy, lean, attractive body. Add to

this winning combination the right supplements and you will achieve

your goals even faster.

For each of the first three cycles of the 6-Pack Prescription, I rec-

ommend specific supplements designed to maximize your results for

that cycle. As I've said earlier, supplements are not essential to my pro-

gram, but they can certainly help enhance your results and accelerate

your progress. For many people, the supplements that I recommend will

provide the boost needed to go from good to great.

In the interest of full disclosure, I do have to note that, as many readers already know, I have designed the Body Rx: 6-Pack Prescription line of supplements. However, I am presenting my supplement plan in generic terms so that you can obtain the supplements from whatever source you find most economical and convenient.

For Cycle 1: Get Stronger
Creatine Monohydrate

Creatine monohydrate is an amino acid found in meat and fish. Since it hit the market in 1993, creatine has become the most popular sports supplement of all time, used by millions of professional athletes and weekend warriors. Creatine is the perfect supplement for Cycle 1 for one simple reason: It helps build strength. In fact, studies show that taking creatine can increase strength by about 10 percent, helping to build the foundation you need for a better body. Creatine provides more fuel to muscle cells, allowing them to work harder and you to get better results in the gym. It helps you recharge your muscles between sets so that you can get the most out of your body. It won't magically make you stronger if you don't work out, but if you do, it can enhance the effect of my weight-lifting regimen. Fast-twitch muscle fibers, the kind used to handle short-term, heavy-duty workloads like weight lifting, have the highest concentrations of creatine.

Creatine is extremely well documented. In fact, there have been more than 300 studies on it, most of them overwhelmingly positive. Creatine is a hot seller because it works, and I think that it can work for you.

Creatine monohydrate is added to some protein powders and is also sold separately as a powder or in capsules. For those who are taking protein supplements, it makes sense to use one that contains creatine during this cycle.

For days 1 to 10, you will take 10 grams of creatine daily. If you choose to purchase your creatine separately, simply mix 10 grams of creatine powder in a glass of unsweetened fruit juice. Creatine is best absorbed when taken with both protein and carbohydrates, so take your creatine when you eat a meal or add protein powder to the creatine juice mixture.

For the rest of Cycle 1, cut back to 5 grams of creatine each day.

Cycle 2: Get Sculpted
HMB

HMB (short for b-hydroxy-b-methylbutyrate) is a substance that is naturally produced in the body from foods containing leucine, an amino acid. HMB is tailor made to complement the exercise program in Cycle 2, enhancing your efforts at the gym. HMB appears to have a protein-sparing effect. In other words, it reduces protein loss during exercise so that more protein is available to build muscle. Studies have shown that HMB can increase strength and muscle size by as much as 250 percent—not a bad result when your goal for this cycle is to build up your muscle mass. HMB does a lot of other good things for your body as well, including lowering LDL (low-density lipoprotein) or "bad" cholesterol.

HMB is safe; there are no known side effects. In fact, it's being investigated as a medical treatment for wasting syndrome in cancer patients.

Take 3 grams of HMB daily. HMB is an ingredient in some protein powders and bars and is also available separately in capsule form. You can simplify your supplement regimen by using an HMB-enriched protein powder or bar during this cycle, or take three 1,000-mg capsules daily with food.

For Cycle 3: Burn Fat
Green Tea

Green tea, popular in Asia, is a less processed form of the black tea commonly drunk in the West. Many of you already know that green tea may protect against different forms of cancer and heart disease. What you may not know is that a chemical found in green tea shows signs of being a potent fat burner. Scientists suspect that an antioxidant found in green tea, epigallocatechin gallate (EGCG), is the chemical that turns up your body's fat-burning furnaces—not the caffeine, as was commonly thought. A study published in the *American Journal of Clinical Nutrition* reported that capsules containing the amount of EGCG in about 2 to 3 cups of green tea can increase the amount of energy burned over a twenty-four-hour period by about 4 percent. More important, the study reported that EGCG enhanced fat burning by about 10 percent. Rather than flood you with green tea, I recommend taking a supplement. It's much easier to do.

Green tea is available in capsules. Take three 250-mg capsules daily. Look for green tea extract standardized to 75 percent catechins, containing 50 percent epigallocatechin gallate.

DIM

DIM (Diidolymethane) is a chemical derived from cruciferous vegetables such as broccoli, cauliflower, cabbage, and Brussels sprouts. When you eat these vegetables, DIM is formed during digestion. DIM is an important hormone regulator. It alters the breakdown of the female hormone estrogen so that there are fewer cancer-causing estrogens and more of the good, health-promoting variety. In the process of controlling bad estrogens, DIM metabolites are processed by the same enzyme systems that break down an important fat-burning hormone called epinephrine. Epinephrine is critical for body composition because it controls the release of fatty acids from fat cells. The more epinephrine, the more fat you will burn. In the process of altering estrogen metabolism, DIM helps preserve circulating levels of epinephrine, enhancing fat burning.

Why should guys worry about estrogen? In men, excess estrogen can have a detrimental effect on body composition, contributing to abdominal obesity (that annoying spare tire) and increasing the risk of prostate cancer. DIM may help maintain the level of free testosterone, which helps balance excess estrogen. Given all that we know of DIM's positive effect on hormone balance, I believe that it will enhance the fat-burning phase, particularly in combination with green tea and MCTs.

Women: Take one 75-mg capsule of DIM daily.

Men: Take two 75-mg capsules daily.

Medium-Chain Triglycerides

Eat fat to lose fat? It works, as long as it's the right kind of fat. Medium-chain triglycerides (MCTs) are a special kind of fatty acid derived from coconut and palm kernel oil. Smaller than the longer-chain fatty acids normally found in most other fats and oils, MCTs bypass the normal digestive process and are rapidly absorbed by the body. When given the option, the body will burn MCTs for energy over protein and glucose, which both spares protein (to make more lean mass) and stimulates more fat loss, precisely your goals for Cycle 3. MCTs are hardly new: They have been used for 30 years to enhance athletic performance, promote weight loss, and treat medical problems relating to the absorption of longer-chain fatty acids.

MCT oil can be purchased at most health food stores and even some supermarkets. MCT is also an added ingredient in some protein powders and bars. MCTs should not be used in cooking, as they have a lower melting point than long-chain fatty acids, and will burn at lower temperatures. (MCTs may cause stomach upset in some people, so it's wise to gradually increase your intake, and don't use them on an empty stomach. MCTs in protein powders or bars are easier to digest and should not cause any GI problems.)

During the fat-burning phase, I recommend that you add MCT oil to your protein shake, or use a protein powder or bar that already contains MCT. During the first week of this cycle, add 1 teaspoon of MCT oil twice a day; for Week 2, add 2 teaspoons twice a day and for Weeks 3 to 6, add 1 tablespoon of oil twice daily.

MY 6-PACK PRESCRIPTION SUPPLEMENT CHART

Cycle	Supplements	Daily Guidelines
1 Getting Stronger	Creatine Monohydrate	**Days 1–10:** 10 grams a day taken with protein and carbohydrates **Days 11–42:** 5 grams a day taken with protein and carbohydrates **Note:** It's easiest to take your creatine in the form of a protein shake fortified with creatine monohydrate. Or you can mix creatine powder into a glass of juice.
2 Getting Sculpted	HMB	3 grams a day **Note:** Some protein shakes and bars are enriched with HMB, but be sure to get enough. HMB is also available in capsule form. Take three 1,000-mg capsules a day with food.
3 Burning Fat	Green Tea	Three 250-mg capsules a day, standardized to 50% catechins, containing 75% epigallocatechin gallate (EGCG)
	DIM	**Men:** One 75-mg capsule a day **Women:** Two 75-mg capsules a day
	MCT	**Week 1:** One teaspoon twice a day **Week 2:** Two teaspoons twice a day **Weeks 3–6:** One tablespoon twice a day **Note:** MCTs are easiest to get and digest in a protein shake or bar.

9

Body R_x: Women

Although I am writing this chapter for women, I want to make one important point before I go any further. Nature did not intend for one sex to be strong and muscular, and the other sex to be weak and flabby. Nature did not intend for one sex to eat food and the other sex to starve. The principles of fitness and nutrition do not change according to gender. The program outlined in *Body Rx* is perfect for a woman's body. Whether you are a man or a woman, if you follow the 6-Pack Prescription, I promise that you will achieve great results.

This is not to say that women do not have specific concerns. However, women need not eat or work out differently from how men do.

On the contrary, in this chapter I intend to convince you that women should be doing *exactly* the same thing as men. I understand that many women may be resistant to the idea that they should eat six meals a day and lift weights. They have been socialized to believe that those activities are the province of men. Moreover, too many women are convinced that food is the enemy and subscribe to the prevailing myth that weight lifting will make them big and masculine. In fact, just the opposite is true! Eating the right food, and lots of it, will slim you down. Following my weight-training program will give you a sculpted, beautiful, and smaller body.

Women often confuse weight training with bodybuilding. I've done both, and believe me, they are worlds apart. A bodybuilder—male or female—is seeking to create the largest musculature that they can. Weight training, by contrast, aims to make you fit, firm, and healthy. If you want the kind of sculpted, lovely body that you've always dreamed about, weight training and proper nutrition are not the enemy: They are your best weapon. I'm not asking you to give up your femininity, just your fat!

In many ways, women stand to benefit even more from my program than men. From their teenage years on, women have been the primary victims of our diet-obsessed culture. Women have been conditioned to believe that it is virtuous to skip meals and starve themselves. Most women spend their lives on weight-loss diets and still don't like the way they look. The problem is, they are locked in a losing battle with their bodies. Everything they are doing is working against their metabolism, creating a metabolic meltdown that ruins their bodies and their lives. The 6-Pack Prescription liberates women from destructive behaviors such as counting calories, skipping meals out of fear of gaining weight, and doing aerobics till they're blue (or red) in the face. Women torture themselves this way and *still* don't like the way they look and feel.

Muscle Is a Woman's Issue

My message to women is this: *Stop focusing on losing weight and start focusing on making muscle.* Muscle is what makes your body look sexy and trim. Fat is what makes you look flabby and unattractive. And muscle is what burns your fat off—not restrictive dieting, not endless aerobics, not trying to shrink yourself down to nothing. The inability of women to build enough muscle when they are young, and the rapid loss of muscle when they are old, are the number-one threats to women's health. This leads to devastating health problems in the long term and brutally restrictive regimens and yo-yo dieting in the short term.

Many physical trainers have told me how frustrated they are with their women clients because they don't come close to reaching their full physical potential. Many women are reluctant to work out with the correct intensity in the mistaken belief that they are not built to be strong. Trust me: Nature intended for women to be strong! It amazes me that women who refuse to lift more than 5- or 10-pound weights at the gym (or to lift weights at all!) don't realize how much weight they actually must lift in real-life situations. You need strong muscles to pick up a 40-pound toddler, or haul a 20-pound bag of groceries, or even carry a pregnancy to term without suffering constant backaches. If you don't have adequate muscle, you are more likely to sustain an injury.

The irony is, when women do begin to work out, they are often surprised by their innate strength. When it comes to weight lifting, women actually make faster progress than men, and in fact often have lower-body strength that is proportionally equal to that of men. Although women typically have less upper-body strength than men due to less muscle mass, they can still make tremendous strides in terms of increasing their strength and improving their appearance. There is no reason for any woman to have hunched-over shoulders due to weak muscles or flabby, unconditioned upper arms! Weight training is the cure for these common cosmetic problems that can lead to severe medical problems down the road.

The problem is, women do not build the underlying muscle that is necessary to maintain their bodies because they do not exercise correctly. Look around you at the gym. Women using the aerobics equipment outnumber the women in the weight room by 10:1. When women do lift weights, they tend to lift very light weights without progressing properly to the next stage. There's no *work* in their workout! Aerobics and light lifting do not make new muscle or help preserve existing muscle. If you starve yourself and do these things, sure, you'll get thin, but you won't get lean. Moreover, you'll be in a constant battle with yourself to maintain that illusory thinness. Without muscle, you can't burn enough body fat, and you'll still be flabby. Flabby "thin/fat" young women turn into weak/fat old women, and that can have tragic repercussions.

Muscle is the engine that drives metabolism. The more muscle you have, the more fat you burn. The converse is also true: The less muscle you have, the more fat you will store. The more fat you store, the more likely you are to become obese. For women, obesity greatly increases the odds of becoming diabetic, having a heart attack, getting colon or breast cancer, or developing any number of serious illnesses.

A lifetime of dieting can wreak havoc on a woman's body. The standard low-calorie, high-carbohydrate, low-protein diet is not one that will help you make muscle or maintain muscle. It is one that will create metabolic aberrations that will ultimately make you fatter despite your best efforts to stay thin. When you go on a low-calorie diet, you don't just lose fat: One third of your weight loss is muscle. If you go off the diet and gain the weight back, those new pounds are 80 percent fat and only 20 percent muscle. The more you yo-yo up and down the scale, the more muscle you destroy and the more fat you gain.

The human body was not designed to go hungry. When you don't give your body the food it needs, when it needs it, it protects itself by conserving energy. In other words, it tries to store as much fat as possible. When you combine inadequate calories with a lack of protein, you compound an already bad situation. Without enough protein, your body does not have enough amino acids on hand to do all its important work. Your body runs on amino acids, after all. To make up the shortfall, your body robs amino acids from your muscles. That's why dieting burns off muscle more than fat. In that kind of environment, you gradually deplete your muscle tissue and growing new muscle is an absolute impossibility. This can be catastrophic to women.

As women age, hormone changes produce a natural, gradual decline in muscle mass. Because of this, women are at great risk of becoming sarcopenic—that is, severely deficient in muscle. People who suffer from wasting syndrome are sarcopenic; ironically, so are many obese women. You need muscle mass to generate the metabolic engine to burn off your body fat, and sarcopenic women don't have enough. They just get fatter and fatter and fatter until they are so burdened by their body mass that they can barely move—can barely breathe. Because it has become so difficult to walk even a few steps, these women become totally inactive, making their condition even worse. Ironically, many of these women are put on the typical low-calorie, high-carb, low-protein diets by their doctors in the hope of causing weight loss. As you know by now, that only makes them fatter. Up until a few years ago, it was rare to see a truly sarcopenic women, but today they are everywhere. You'll notice that these women are often in wheelchairs, not for any injury or physical impairment, but because they don't have enough muscle to hold up their frames. It must be a miserable way to grow old.

Cellulite: The Toughest Fat of All

The most common complaint that I hear from women about their bodies is "I have cellulite, and I hate it!" Cellulite is the popular term used to describe fatty deposits around the hips, buttocks, and thighs. Men don't get cellulite, but when they do have extra fat, they tend to carry it around their abdomens, not their lower bodies. Since women are the ones who get pregnant, nature wanted to ensure that even when the food supply was scarce, women had a fighting chance of delivering a healthy baby. As a result of hormone receptor differences between men and women, women hold on to more fat than men do, especially around the hips, buttocks, and thighs. In the past, women may have needed these fat deposits during difficult times, but today, when food is abundant and the birth rate is low, cellulite has become the nemesis of many women. No one has ever taken a poll, but I'm willing to bet that cellulite is the number-one reason why women hate putting on a bathing suit. Some so-called experts will tell you that cellulite is different from regular fat, and that nothing short of surgical removal can remove it. The reality is, cellulite deposits are just fat cells, but of a particularly stubborn variety. As most women already know, fat deposits on the lower body are more resistant to fat burning than other fat cells. Nevertheless, you can get rid of cellulite, but you have to be very careful how you do it.

Going on a low-calorie diet is the worst thing you can do. It will only aggravate the situation by making your fat cells even more determined than ever to protect you from the impending famine.

The 6-Pack Prescription Meal Plan is a terrific way to encourage fat loss everywhere in the body—even those areas riddled with cellulite. Protein and fiber will help liberate fat from those reluctant areas, but weight training will move things along faster. My weight-training program is a particularly effective way to break up cellulite deposits. As I discussed in Chapter 8, epinephrine, the hormone that is controlled by the central nervous system, is instrumental in the release of fatty acids from fat cells. Weight training makes fat cells more sensitive to epinephrine, which can turn up fat burning. In addition, the process of weight training creates muscle—the new metabolic engine to burn even more fat. I'm not saying that getting rid of cellulite is easy, but it's not impossible. (Women may also benefit from DIM, a supplement that promotes fat burning. See page 254.)

Muscle Protects Bones

One out of four women (as compared to one out of six men) will get osteoporosis, the thinning or wearing away of bones that increases susceptibility to breaks. Areas that are particularly vulnerable include the vertebrae, hips, and forearms. Losing some bone is a natural part of the aging process. At around age 30, people develop their peak bone mass. A slowing down in the production of new bone then sets in, and after age 30, people begin to lose about 1 percent of their bone mass each year. After menopause, women begin to lose between 2 and 4 percent of their bone mass each year for about a decade until it levels off. This bone loss has real consequences. A significant number of all postmenopausal women in the U.S. will suffer vertebral fractures, which can lead to the unsightly dowager's hump or rounded back. Osteoporosis is not just a cosmetic issue: It can be life-threatening. One out of six older women will break a hip sometime in her lifetime, and 20 percent will die of complications from that injury, notably infection. (For further explanation on the relationship of protein to the high mortality rate from injury among the elderly, see Chapter 10.)

Women need to take steps to protect themselves against osteoporosis early in life. Good nutrition is key. The process of making and repairing bone requires the right mix of protein, vitamins, and minerals. Women who are constantly on low-calorie diets may not be getting enough of these nutrients in their food. Both men and women need to be concerned about consuming enough calcium, the mineral that is essential for bone growth. I recommend that both men and women try to get about 2,000 mg of calcium daily; 1,000 mg from food and another 1,000 mg from calcium supplements. In fact, the complete meal replacement protein supplements that I recommend contain almost a day's worth of calcium in one serving. Low-fat or nonfat cottage cheese and nonfat yogurt are also good sources of calcium.

Weight training can slow down bone loss as well as increase muscle mass. Strong muscles can protect bones and joints from injury. Strong muscles also keep you steadier on your feet, which will help prevent injuries in the first place. And strong muscles will keep you from becoming the proverbial hunched-over "little old woman."

If you already have osteoporosis, weight training can help prevent further bone loss, but you need to check with your doctor first to see if there are any exercises that you should not do because of the increased risk of fractures. The earlier you catch osteoporosis, the better; with the right diet and workout routine, you can stop the problem before it becomes too severe. Women with severe osteoporosis should talk to their physicians about hormone replacement therapy after menopause, which may also help slow down bone loss.

Invest in Yourself

I know that women today are laden with family and work responsibilities, leaving little time for themselves. Many are under a great deal of stress and find it understandably difficult to juggle their numerous roles. When you're overwhelmed by so many different demands, there's a tendency to put your own needs last. You may think that you are benefiting others by denying yourself, but in reality you are not. Making time for yourself is not being selfish; it's being smart. If you don't keep yourself in good physical condition, you cannot function optimally at work or be there for your family at home. If you're careless about what you eat, and if you don't get to the gym, you will not have the energy or the stamina to fulfill your many different jobs. If you don't take care of yourself, you won't feel well, you won't feel good about how you look, and your negative feelings will spill over into other aspects of your life. Nor will you be setting a good example for your family! Kids learn from their parents. If you set fitness and health as a priority, they will follow your example.

It is my hope that the 6-Pack Prescription will change the way women think about their bodies and themselves. In the future, when women talk about their weight, they'll be talking about the weights they lift at the gym, not what the scale says. In the future, when women think about food, they'll be thinking about all the protein and fiber they need to eat that day, and not trying to be sure they eat as little as possible. Finally, in the future, when women look at themselves in the mirror, they'll be thinking, *I look strong, sculpted, and lean, and I plan on staying that way for the rest of my life.*

10

It's Never Too Late

When you hear someone say the words "old person," what image

pops into your head?

Do you see a frail, weak, hunched-over man or woman creeping

along with a cane or walker? Do you see someone who is confined by

physical debility and who is growing progressively weaker with each

passing year?

That's not the image that I see when I think of an old person. When

I think of an old person, I think of people at my gym who are in their

sixties and seventies (and maybe even older) who lift weights side by side

with younger people and have lean, attractive bodies that could put some 30-year-olds to shame! I see grandmas and grandpas who don't wrench their back every time they swoop down to give their grandkids a hug, who can still play a killer game of tennis, and who are still enjoying rich, full, healthy lives.

Given a choice, wouldn't you rather be the kind of old person that I envision than the stereotypical sickly older person held hostage by a body that is falling apart? My Body Rx program gives you that choice.

In recent years it's become popular to talk about the "diseases of aging" as if they are inevitable. Indeed, some scientists refer to aging itself as a disease. I'm sorry, but that's nonsense! The sickly, weak, hunched-over "old" person is not a true reflection of natural aging: It's the result of decades of poor nutrition, neglect, and sitting idly by while bones crumble and muscles vanish. With proper nutrition, exercise, and adequate muscle, the human body can remain vital and strong well into the last decades of life. I'm living proof that muscle keeps you young. At 50 years old, I'm in better shape than most 20-year-olds and I intend to stay that way. In fact, I'm in the best shape of my life!

But old prejudices die hard. There is still a popular misconception that the gym is the domain of the young, and that no matter how hard an older person may work out, he or she can't reverse the ravages of time. Not true!

Fitness is not the exclusive domain of the young. At any age, you can be vital and strong. At any age, you can get stronger, sculpted, and leaner from my program. If you are in good health and do not have any specific physical problems, regardless of your age, you can follow the 6-Pack Prescription Meal Plan and weight-training regimen. My meal plan in particular is ideal for older people because it will help prevent the common metabolic diseases, such as diabetes, heart disease, and nutritional deficiencies, that run rampant among the older population.

My workout regimen is also ideal for older people, but here I must add a few caveats. If you are middle-aged or older and have never worked out before, there are a few extra precautions that you need to take. The older you are, the greater the possibility that you may have an undiagnosed medical problem such as heart disease or arthritic joints or other structural weakness that could be aggravated by the wrong exercise. *Therefore, it is imperative for you to have a thorough physical examination before you begin any workout regimen.* If you do have a physical problem, it doesn't mean that you can't work out, but you may have to work around it. It is particularly important for you to work with a knowledgeable trainer who can help prevent injuries.

I want to stress that even though you may be in your later decades, your workout strategy should be the same as a younger person. In order to achieve good results, you need to work out with enough intensity to make a difference in your body. Obviously, if you are so frail that you can't walk without the aid of a walker or a cane, the intensity of your workout will be different from that of a peer who has weight trained all his or her life and who is still in great shape. But don't let age or physical debility discourage you. Studies of older people have shown that a good weight-training regimen can greatly enhance strength and stability in people as old as 100! In other words, it's never too late to benefit from my program.

There is no natural reason why aging should be synonymous with frailty, debility, and disease. In fact, it's nature's plan for you to be robust until the very end. As I mentioned in Chapter 2, we humans are the only large mammals that progressively lose muscle strength, grow frail, and get sicker with each passing decade. Our caveman ancestors managed to retain muscle mass and bone strength well into old age. And so can we, despite our longer life spans. The key, as you've probably guessed by now, is muscle.

Muscle Loss: The Real "Disease" of Aging

The number-one health problem of aging is not cancer, heart disease, osteoporosis, or one of the so-called diseases of aging. The number-one problem of aging is the loss of muscle mass. Starting around 30, we lose 2 to 4 pounds of muscle every decade, which can add up to a huge loss of muscle by the time we hit our sixth or seventh decade. The typical 65-year old has 20 pounds less lean mass than when he or she was 25! The loss of muscle not only makes us weaker and flabbier but has a profound effect on all aspects of our health and life.

Most people hope that they can spend their last decades of life living independent, active lives; yet, many are forced to retreat into nursing homes or long-term care facilities. Why? If you think that most people are in nursing homes because they are sick or are suffering from diminished mental function, you're wrong. Most people are in nursing homes for one simple reason: They don't have the muscle strength to lift themselves out of a chair without assistance or to walk around on their own. Their muscles have grown so weak, they can't even withstand the normal forces of gravity. The loss of mobility prevents people from doing everyday tasks that keep them independent, like shopping, cooking, and even bathing. Surely, this could not be what nature intended for us.

The loss of muscle can also have a profoundly negative impact on cardiovascular function. Remember, your heart is also a muscle. Weight training can strengthen your heart muscle just as it strengthens other muscles in your body. When you work against resistance, such as when you are lifting a weight, it forces your heart to pump harder, which produces thicker, stronger walls. The stronger your heart, the easier it will be for it to do its job. At one time, heart patients were discouraged from doing weight training in the mistaken belief that it raised blood pressure and placed undue stress on the heart. Today, cardiologists know that just the opposite is true. A sedentary lifestyle actually increases your risk of developing heart disease, and a well-designed workout regimen can help maintain a healthy heart. (Of course, if you have a preexisting heart condition, you must talk to your doctor before embarking on any exercise regimen. Your doctor may recommend a training facility that is affiliated with a hospital or medical center where you will be well supervised.)

Muscle wasting not only exacts a steep toll on individuals, it comes with a steep price tag. Medical costs have skyrocketed in recent years as the population ages. Today there are 35 million Americans over the age of 65, but in 2030 there will be 70 million. If we don't take steps to change the "normal" course of aging—if we end up with tens of millions of people in their seventies and eighties who can't get up out of their chairs—society will be bankrupted by the cost of caring for them. There's a simple, inexpensive solution to this problem: the 6-Pack Prescription.

Protein: The Anti-Aging Nutrient

I believe that much of the muscle loss that has become synonymous with aging can be prevented through a lifetime of proper nutrition, and in particular by eating enough protein. Throughout this book I've touted the fat-burning, muscle-building properties of protein, but I want you to understand that protein is not just a "diet" food. It is a powerful anti-aging nutrient.

Protein is the body's primary source of amino acids. We've been taught to think of amino acids as the building blocks of protein and little else, but in fact, they are the building blocks of life itself. You can't make or maintain muscle without amino acids, which are stored primarily in muscle cells. Amino acids help regulate blood pressure, turn genes on and off, and run the brain. Amino acids are critical to a man's ability to achieve and maintain an erection.

Amino acids play an especially critical role in the running of the immune system. Among all amino acids, glutamine is one of the most important for a well-functioning immune system. Glutamine is one of the most abundant amino acids in the body, and most of the glutamine used by the body is obtained from glutamine stores in muscle. Without enough glutamine, you cannot launch a successful attack against a serious infection or maintain your muscles.

What if you don't get enough amino acids in your diet to cover all your needs? Your body compensates for the deficiency by diverting amino acids from body stores, primarily from muscle, to another location in your body that needs them the most. For example, you get sick and need extra glutamine to make more immune cells. Your immune system grabs what it needs from your muscles, creating a relative drain that subsequently leads to serious disturbances in the functional balance of other amino acids as well. As a result, you become fat and flabby. This is precisely what happens as we age.

If the intake of protein is low for a long period of time, as it is for so many people following the typical high-carbohydrate diet, protein reserves are depleted and the results can be deadly. Not only are you cheating your body out of its daily supply of amino acids, but you have progressively robbed your muscle tissue of them as well. Hence a critical protein reserve component is progressively diminished. When you lose muscle, not only are you losing your storehouse of available amino acids, you're losing your lifeline.

Take, for example, an elderly woman who fractures a hip, an injury that should not be life threatening. Yet, 20 percent of all women who fracture their hips die within six months. Why? These women don't die of their injuries; they die of infections such as pneumonia. I think the real cause of death is functional protein deficiency. Let me explain why. As I'm sure you recall, the immune system runs on amino acids. When you suffer an injury, your immune system is sent into overdrive to keep the body healthy as it heals. But what if you have a low-protein diet and don't have enough muscle to maintain an adequate reserve of amino acids? Your body will rapidly deplete your amino acid reserve, your immune system will be compromised, and, sadly, the end result is death. I believe that much of this disaster can be offset by maintaining a lifetime of optimal protein intake.

As we age, we need even more amino acids to repair and replenish worn old cells—not the opposite, as is so often preached. Some experts argue that as people get older, they should eat less protein because they're not as active as they used to be. I think that's just wrong. Older people who are poorly nourished will have even less energy and lose more muscle! That will make them even less likely to engage in activities that help to enhance appetite and build up muscle. So they grow frailer and weaker.

Poor nutrition, and in particular an inadequate intake of protein, poses a real health threat among older people. Precisely at a time when their bodies need protein the most, they tend to cut back on food. The "thin/fat" phenomenon that I described earlier not only occurs in young, chronic dieters, but is a special problem among the old. Even though they may be very thin due to a reduction in food intake, older people are often not lean. Decades of poor eating habits and inactivity have chewed up their muscle and lean mass, leaving them thin yet flabby. The problem is only exacerbated with age because an older person who is not active may not get as hungry as a younger person and may end up skipping meals. For many older people, eating six smaller meals daily is easier than the standard three large meals and is far better in terms of providing a constant flow of amino acids. Protein shakes are another great way for older people to keep their protein intake at optimal levels. Many older people are already drinking meal-replacement beverages, but those marketed specifically to the elderly tend not to be as good a source of protein as the standard protein powders and ready-to-drink protein beverages that I recommend. There's no reason why older people should not use the same protein supplements as younger people.

Grow Young at the Gym

If you want to reclaim your body, there is no better place to do it than at the gym. Regardless of your age or physical condition, you can benefit from weight training. Weight training is the only way to preserve muscle, make new muscle, and increase bone mass. Until recently, most older people were steered away from the gym by experts who believed that weight training was too strenuous an activity for seniors. "Stay out of the gym," they warned. "You'll just get hurt. If you want to exercise, try walking! Remember the mantra 'Walking is the best exercise'?"

Turns out these so-called experts were dead wrong. Walking may be a great mode of transportation, but it does little to improve your body. And ironically, for older people with poor muscle strength, walking may be dangerous to their health. People who are so weak that they are unsteady on their feet are more likely to fall while walking, which could lead to broken bones. Complications from injuries due to broken bones are a leading cause of death among the elderly. And by the way, the vast majority of these accidents don't occur at the gym: They occur right in people's own homes doing everyday tasks like walking up stairs or bathing!

The experts are beginning to change their tune. Recent studies have shown that people as old as 100 can benefit from weight training:

- A study conducted at the USDA Human Nutrition Research Center on Aging at Tufts University showed that a high-intensity, lower-body strength-training program more than doubled muscle strength in frail, older people ages 86 to 90.

None of the subjects suffered injury. Weight training also improved their balance and walking speed.

- When older men (ages 65 to 70) did weight-training exercises at the same intensity as younger men, their muscle fibers increased in size at the same rate as those of younger exercisers. Similar to younger exercisers, their muscle fibers also changed from being poor fat burners to being champion fat burners.

- Numerous studies have documented that weight training can increase bone density in older people, which can help prevent osteoporosis, the thinning of bone, making it vulnerable to breaks.

- A study of people living in a nursing home showed that after completing a strength-training program, they were more likely to engage in social activities and eat in a communal dining room rather than alone in their rooms. Why? They were better able to move around on their own. In fact, the researchers were so impressed by the results that they surmised that if more of these older people had participated in strength-training programs, they might have been able to avoid the kinds of falls and injuries that forced them into the nursing home in the first place.

Muscle strength can make the difference between being confined to a life of isolation and loneliness because of physical frailty and being able to move freely in society without fear that you will fall with every step you take, or that you will sit down and not be able to stand up again. I am so passionate about getting older people to the gym that I think every Medicare card should come with a lifetime gym membership!

There is no reason why you can't follow the 6-Pack Prescription workout plan with some modifications based on your medical history. For example, if you have an arthritic knee or a back problem, you may need to adjust a few of the exercises to work for you, but you can still perform many of the same exercises. Remember, at any age, the same rules of muscle building apply: You need to work your muscles hard enough to get results. If you lift too light, you're wasting your time (and money, if you're paying a trainer). Then again, if you lift too heavy, you can injure yourself, especially if you have an underlying structural problem. An experienced trainer will help you work out at the right level for you. I want to caution older people against buying a set of free weights and trying to work out on their own at home. Working at the gym on machines is actually safer because machines limit your range of motion and make injury less likely.

I know some older people may be put off at the thought of walking into a gym. You may think that you're going to stick out like a sore thumb. Not so: You'd be surprised how many people in their sixties, seventies, and beyond are now working out. In fact, many gyms cater to an older population, and you should try to find one in your area that will accommodate your needs.

The benefits of the 6-Pack Prescription extend far beyond looking great in a bathing suit, or feeling gratified that you can get through the day with energy to spare. My program enables you to grow older in a body that stays younger. The title of this chapter, "It's Never Too Late," reflects my own belief in the power of the 6-Pack Prescription. Whatever your age or physical condition, better nutrition and the right workout regimen can make a profound change in your life—not just for now, but for decades to come.

Ascherio, A., Willet, W.C., "Health Effects of Transfatty Acids." *Am J Clin Nutr* 66 (suppl) (1997), 1006S–1010S.

Bach, A., et al. Medium-chain Triglycerides: An Update." *Am J Clin Nutr* 36 (1982), 990–962.

Bantle, J.P., et al. "Effects of Dietary Fructose on Plasma Lipids in Healthy Subjects." *Am J Clin Nutr* 72 (2000), 1128–1134.

Bouchard, C., et al. "The Response to Long Term Overfeeding in Identical Twins." *New England Journal of Medicine* 322:21 (May 24, 1990), 1477–1482.

Daly, M.E., et al. "Dietary Carbohydrate and Insulin Sensitivity: A Review of the Evidence and Clinical Implications." *Amer J Clin Nutr* 66 (1997), 1072–1085.

Dangin, M., et al. "The Digestion Rate of Protein is an Independent Regulating Factor of Postprandial Protein Retention." *Am J Physiol Endocrinol Metab* 280 (2001), E340–348.

Demling, R.H., et al. "Increased Protein Intake During the Recovery Phase After Severe Burns Increases Body Weight Gain and Muscle Function." *Journal of Burn Care and Rehabilitation* 19:2 (1998), 161–168.

Demling, R. "Effect of a Hypocaloric Diet, Increased Protein Intake and Resistance Training on Lean Mass Gains and Fat Mass Loss in Overweight Police Officers." *Annals of Nutrition and Metabolism* 44 (2000), 21–29.

Dirlewanger, M., et al. "Effects of Fructose on Hepatic Glucose Metabolism in Humans." *Am J Physiol Endocrinol Metab* 279 (2000), E911.

Dulloo, A.G. "Efficacy of a Green Tea Extract Rich in Catechin Polyphenols and Caffeine in Increasing 24-Hour Energy Expenditure and Fat Oxidation in Humans." *Am J Clin Nutr* 70 (1999), 1040–1045.

Eaton, S.B., Eaton, S.B. III, Konner, M.J., et al. "An Evolutionary Perspective Enhances Understanding of Human Nutritional Requirements." *Journal of Nutrition* 126 (1996), 1732–1740.

Eaton, S.B., et al., "Paleolithic Nutrition Revisited: A Twelve Year Retrospective on its Nature and Implications." *European Journal of Clinical Nutrition* 51 (1997), 207–216.

Fiatarone, M., et al., "Exercise Training and Nutritional Supplementation for Physical Frailty in Very Elderly People." *New England Journal of Medicine* 25 (June 23, 1994), 1769–1775.

Fordslund, A.H., et al. "Effect of Protein Intake and Physical Activity on 24-H Pattern and Rate of Micronutrient Utilization." *Amer Physiol Soc* (1999), E964–E976.

Hallfrisch, H. "Metabolic Effects of Dietary Fructose." *The FASEB Journal* 4 (1990), 2652–2660.

Hudgins, L. "Effect of High-Carbohydrate Feeding on Triglyceride and Saturated Fatty Acid Synthesis." *Proc. Soc for Exp Biol Med* (2000), 225: 178–183.

Hudgins, L., et al. "Relationship Between Carbohydrate Induced Hypertriglyceridemia and Fatty Acid Synthesis in Lean and Obese Subjects." *Journal of Lipid Research* 41 (2000), 595–604.

Hunter, G., et al. "Resistance Training Increases Total Energy Expenditure and Free-Living Physical Activity in Older Adults." *J Appl Physiol* 89 (2000), 977–984.

James, W.P.T., et al. "Nutrient Partitioning," in *Handbook of Obesity*, edited by George A. Bray, Claude Bouchard, and W.P.T. James. New York: Marcel Dekker, Inc. (1997), 555–571.

Jeppeson, J., et al. "Postprandial Triglyceride and Retinyl Ester Responses to Oral Fat: Effect of Fructose." *Am J Clin Nutr* 61 (1995), 781–791.

Knopp, R.H. "One-year Effects of Increasingly Fat-Restricted, Carbohydrate Enriched Diets on Lipoprotein Levels in Free-Living Subjects." *Proc Soc Exp Biol Med* (2000), 225:191–199.

Kraemer, W.J., et al. "Effects of Heavy-Resistance Training on Hormonal Response Patterns in Younger vs. Older Men." *J of Appl Physiol* (1999), 982–992.

Lee, B.M., et al. "Effects of Glucose, Sucrose and Fructose on Plasma Glucose and Insulin Responses in Normal Humans: Comparison with White Bread." *European Journal of Clinical Nutrition* 52 (1998), 924–928.

Lemon, P.W.R. "Is Increased Dietary Protein Necessary or Beneficial for Individuals with a Physically Active Lifestyle?" *Nutrition Reviews* 54:4 (1996), S169–175.

Levi, B. et al. "Long Term Fructose Consumption Accelerates Glycation and Several Age-Related Variables in Male Rats." *Journal of Nutrition* 128 (1998), 1442–1449.

Ludwig, D., et al. "Relation Between Consumption of Sugar-Sweetened Drinks and Childhood Obesity." *Lancet* 357:9255 (2001), 505–508.

Ludwig, D., et al. "Dietary Fiber, Weight Grain, and Cardiovascular Disease Risk Factors in Young Adults." *JAMA* 282:16 (1999), 1539–1546.

Mayes, Peter A. "Intermediary Metabolism of Fructose." *Am J Clin Nutr* 58 (suppl) (1993), 754S–765S.

McCrory, M., et al., "Dietary Variety Within Food Groups: Association with Energy Intake and Body Fatness in Men and Women." *Am J Clin Nutr* 69 (1999), 440–447.

Mikkelsen, P., et al. "Effect of Fat-Reduced Diets on 24-H Energy Expenditure: Comparisons Between Animal Protein, Vegetable Protein and Carbohydrate." *Am J Clin Nutr* 72 (2000), 1135–1141.

Millward, D.J. "Metabolic Demands for Amino Acids and the Human Dietary Requirement: Millward and Rivers (1988) Revisited." *J Nutri* (1998), 2563S–2576S.

Mokdad, A.H., et al. "The Spread of the Obesity Epidemic in the United States, 1991–1998." *JAMA* 282:16 (1999), 1519–1522.

Nielson, F.H., et al. "Dietary Fructose and Magnesium Affect Macromineral Metabolism in Men." *Proceedings of the North Dakota Academy of Science* 51 (1997), 212.

Newsholme, E.A., et al. "Glutamine Metabolism in Lymphocytes: Its Biochemical, Physiological and Clinical Importance." *Quarterly Journal of Experimental Physiology* 70 (1985), 473–489.

Nissen, S., et al. "Effect of Leucine Metabolite B-Hydroxy B-Methylbutyrate on Muscle Metabolism During Resistance-Exercise Training." *J Appl Physiol* (1995), 2095–2104.

Parks, E.J., and Hellerstein, M. "Carbohydrate-Induced Hypertriacylglycerolemia: A Historical Perspective and Review of the Biological Mechanisms." *Am J Clin Nutr* 71 (2000), 412–433.

Proctor, D.M., et al. "Age-Related Sarcopenia in Humans Is Associated with Reduced Rates of Specific Muscle Proteins." *J Nutri* (1998), 351S–355S.

Reeds, P.J., Hutchens, T.W. "Protein Requirements: From Nitrogen Balance to Functional Impact." *J Nutri* (1994), 1754S–1963S.

Roubenoff, R. "The Pathophysiology of Wasting in the Elderly." *J Nutri* (1999), 256S–259S.

Starc, T.J., et al. "Greater Dietary Intake of Simple Carbohydrate Is Associated with Lower Concentrations of High-Density-Lipoprotein Cholesterol in Hypercholesterolemic Children," *Am J Clin Nutr* 67 (1998), 1147–1154.

Steenge, G.R. "Stimulatory Effect of Insulin on Creatine Accumulation in Human Skeletal Muscle." *J Appl Physiol* (1998), E974–E978.

Stumvoll, M., et al. "Role of Glutamine in Human Carbohydrate Metabolism in Kidney and Other Tissues." *Kidney International* 55 (1999), 778–792.

Tarnopolsky, M.A., et al. "Evaluation of Protein Requirements for Strength Athletes." *J Appl Physiol* (1992), 1986–1995.

Zeligs, M.A., and Connelly, A.S. *All About DIM*. New York: Avery (2000).